While You Diet

REBOOT

The Skinny on Building Health &

Controlling Weight

by

Theodore K. Fenske

MD, FRCPC, FACC, FCCP

Foreword by
Arya Sharma, MD, PHD

4th Floor Press, Inc.
www.4thfloorpress.com

This book contains the Author's opinions, knowledge, and insights based on his clinical experience and research. Always seek the advice of your physician or other qualified health provider with any questions you may have regarding a medical condition.

ISBN 978-1-988993-32-4
eISBN 978-1-988993-33-1
eISBN 978-1-988993-34-8

1st Printing 2012
2nd Printing 2013
3rd Printing 2017
4th Printing (Reboot) 2020
Printed in Canada
www.4thfloorpress.com
cover art by www.istockphoto.com

Dedicated to Tanya Jacqueline Fenske

My favourite cook and confidante

"Many women do noble things, but you surpass them all."

(Proverbs 31:29)

Phyllis,

Here is to Heart
Health!

TKF

About the Author

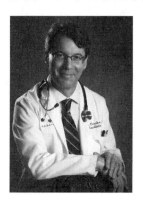

T.K. Fenske is a Clinical Professor with the Division of Cardiology at the University of Alberta, staff cardiologist at the C.K. Hui Heart Centre, Fellow for Medicine and Public Christianity with the Ezra Institute for Contemporary Christianity (EICC), and is an executive member and Chair of the Christian Medical/Dental Association of Canada (CMDA) in Edmonton. He has fellowship training in echocardiography and has formerly been the Principal Teaching Physician at the Royal Alexandra Hospital, and the Director of Cardiac Rehabilitation for the Northern Alberta Program. One of his passions in medicine is the prevention of disease, as evidenced by his speaking involvement in several public forums and his regular written contributions to continuing medical education journals. He is author of *While*

You Quit: a Smoker's Guide to Reducing the Risk of Heart Disease and Stroke (Dundurn ©2009), *While You Diet: The Skinny on Reducing Your Risk of Heart Disease and Stroke* (4th Floor Press ©2012), and *Keeping Faith in Medicine: Navigating Secular Healthcare with Grace and Truth* (Ezra Press ©2020). Formerly from Vancouver, he is the proud father of three sons and content to call Edmonton 'home' where he and his wife, Tanya, are actively involved in the community. In his spare time, Ted enjoys playing guitar, skiing, and running in Edmonton's scenic river valley.

Praise for *While You Diet*

"Waist size matters to your risk for heart disease and stroke. Dr. Fenske, a spokesperson for the Heart and Stroke Foundation, coaches his patients through compelling stories and practical approaches grounded in current research. Understand how you can eat healthy, engage in active living, and reduce your risk—now!" **Donna Hastings, Chief Executive Officer for the Heart and Stroke Foundation of Alberta, NWT & Nunavut**

"At last, a practical guide to eating sensibly—one that can be implemented immediately for a sustained approach to maintaining a decent bodyweight. Written by esteemed Canadian cardiologist, Dr. Ted Fenske, it will prove a worthy companion not only for patients, but also for healthcare professionals working with individuals anxious to look good and feel good, as they battle the challenge of losing weight and keeping it off." **Zaheer Lakhani, MB, ChB, MRCP(UK), FRCPC, FACP, FACC, Professor of Medicine, Order of Canada Recipient 2007**

"It's no surprise Dr. Fenske has delivered another important and accessible book that could help save lives. With his caring and humorous approach, this time Fenske tackles the connections between excess weight and

cardiovascular disease. He provides medical insights mixed with personal anecdotes and explanations that show why we need to maintain a healthy weight for a healthy heart as well as strategies to help us get there." **Donna McElligott, CBC Radio host of Alberta@Noon**

*"What a unique concept! This book takes away from the 'start a diet, stop a diet, or fail at the diet' that so many have struggled with. The day-in-a-life approach will help individuals target problem areas in their lives that can prevent them from leading healthy lifestyles. These tried and true methods, as detailed in **While You Diet**, will be a welcome addition to anyone's bookshelf."* **Maureen Elhatton, Registered Dietician, BSc, BEd, Certified Diabetes Educator, Heart Smart Dietician**

*"This is a very enjoyable and readable book. There are numerous personal and practical perspectives on addressing challenging lifestyle issues, which frustrate weight control. Even the impact on oral health and the possible relationship to cardiovascular problems isn't neglected—a unique insight, which most people would not normally consider. **While You Diet** is an excellent contribution from a distinguished clinician scientist, who actually manages these problems with his patients on a daily basis!"* **Edmund Peters, DDS, MSc, Professor of Dentistry, University of Alberta**

*"**While You Diet** provides important and novel heart-health strategies that can be readily incorporated to improve cardiovascular health and reduce the risk of heart disease and stroke. Given that cardiovascular disease is the leading cause of death worldwide, a finding due in part to obesity, the one-day-at-a-time weight reduction approach in **While You Diet,** focussing on the wider cardiovascular health perspective, is a timely addition to the risk reduction library."* **Mark Haykowsky, PhD, Professor, CIHR New Investigator**

Acknowledgements

With a subject material of this scope, developed over an entire career, it can be a daunting task to know where to begin with thanks and acknowledgements. Fortunately, this isn't my predicament. I have a wonderfully supportive wife to go through life with, including writing this book. Like Bond relies on Q, McCoy leans on Spock, and peanut butter needs jelly, my wife, Tanya, has been my secret weapon, the voice of calm in storms, and added sweetness. She has been my trusty backboard off of which I have bounced ideas over the years and has offered significant behind-the-scenes shaping and editing of this manuscript from its earliest forms. I want to thank her for making it possible for me to have the protected time to tackle this project, which has added an important dimension to my preventative medicine efforts with my patients.

I am very thankful for my cardiology colleagues at the C.K. Hui Heart Institute, for their friendship, abiding support, and commitment to clinical excellence. In particular, I am indebted to the exemplary leadership of our Chief of Cardiology, Dr. Neil Brass, who has calmly steered our division through the challenging waters of administrative restructuring, fiscal restraint, implementation of the behemoth *Connect Care* health information network, and through the problems and panic of the COVID-19 pandemic.

I owe a special thanks to the Cardiac Rehabilitation teams operating in the Edmonton Zone. Their compassionate patient care and keen interest in patient education have been a source of inspiration. I wouldn't have written the first iteration of this book if it hadn't been for the enthusiastic support and encouragement I received from Heather Payette, cardiac rehab nurse extraordinaire. My hope is that this latest edition will continue to enhance the day-to-day clinical engagement of patients in the rehabilitation program and beyond.

I am indebted to the team at 4th Floor Press for their attention to detail, and in particular to Anne Bougie-Johnson for her unfailing encouragement to write this 'reboot edition, her careful review of the manuscript, and untiring commitment to bring this work to timely completion.

Preface for While You Diet
REBOOT

The general reception of *While You Diet* has been a real encouragement for me. In the years following its first publication, I've been delighted to learn how the ideas presented—the analogies, graphs, anecdotes, attempts at humour, and interwoven clinical narrative—have been helpful for my patients, as well as their family members and friends, to both improve their cardiovascular health and assist them with their weight control efforts. However, much has transpired in the world of dieting since that time. As our obesity epidemic has remained unrelenting, and the prevalence of hypertension and diabetes have continued to climb, numerous diets have flooded the market, each promising a remedy to the problematic pounds predicament. From the Keto Diet and Whole 30, to the Alkaline Diet and the Blood-type Diet, and carb cycling, and the Cleanse... and the list goes on and on, a veritable glut of dietary data has landed on our already information-overloaded plates. So, to help sift and sort, and provide some medical perspective, I've updated some of the material in this Reboot edition to address these newer dietary trends, highlighting their merits and underscoring their pitfalls. As well, to provide an easy reference review, each chapter now concludes with a bulleted summary of the key points from the section.

In keeping with the adage, *the more things change, the more things stay the same*, I have continued to emphasize the tried and true heart-healthy dietary approaches. However, while the lion's share of the original manuscript has remained unaltered, there is one noteworthy addition. In this Reboot edition, I've included an approach and rationale for employing strategic intermittent fasting. It's taken some time for me to appreciate the benefits of intermittent fasting, but over recent years, I've been amazed to learn about the myriad benefits of this dietary approach. From enhanced weight control and improvements in glucose regulation, blood pressure and cholesterol lowering, to gastrointestinal health and even longevity, intermittent fasting has been shown to be a valuable adjunct to a healthy lifestyle.[i] This is especially the case when intermittent fasting is added to prudent dietary measures, such as the Pesco-Mediterranean Dietary approach.[ii] So, to address this important, and previously underappreciated dietary discipline (at least to me), I've added a dedicated chapter to review this topic and provide the necessary tools for its safe implementation.

My hope is that this reboot edition of *While You Diet* will encourage and facilitate readers to adopt a sustainable healthy lifestyle. There's just so much to gain from having a regular exercise regimen, choosing whole, unprocessed foods and natural fats, avoiding sugar & refined grains, and balancing restricted feeding with timely fasting. It's widely understood that the majority of chronic illnesses and the development of premature disease could be largely thwarted by such a strategy.[iii] If the COVID-19 pandemic has taught us anything beyond the importance of hand hygiene and social isolation for the elderly and immune-compromised, it's that chronic health liabilities can make us vulnerable to acute health threats. Reviewing the data, it's become apparent that the vast majority of Coronavirus deaths (98 percent) occurred in people with underlying chronic health conditions, such as lung disease, serious heart ailments, obesity, diabetes, chronic kidney disease, and liver disease.[iv] To fortify our immune systems and guard ourselves against infirmity, we need to build and maintain a long-term strategy of health. As Friedrich Nietzsche once said, "the essential thing in heaven and earth… is that there should be long obedience in the same direction."[v] Our health—body, mind, and soul—needs to be approached this way. Appreciating each day as a new one, and seeing each moment and meal as a health opportunity, we would do well to take intentional proven-effective steps to prevent heart disease and stroke, as we build health and control weight.

Theodore K. Fenske, MD, FRCPC, FACC, FCCP
Clinical Professor of Medicine, University of Alberta
Staff Cardiologist, CK Hui Heart Centre
Edmonton, Alberta, Canada

Chapter Notes

i. de Cabo, R. Mattson MP. Effects of Intermittent Fasting on Health, Aging, and Disease. N Engl J Med 2019; 381:2541-2551.

ii: Journal of the American College of Cardiology September 22, 2020, 76 (12) 1484-1493

iii. Prevention of chronic disease in the 21st century: elimination of the leading preventable causes of premature death and disability in the USA. The Lancet July 2014; Volume 384; Issue 9937: pp 45-52.

iv. https://whdh.com/news/nearly-every-mass-coronavirus-death-was-patient-with-underlying-medical-condition-data-shows/

v. Friedrich Nietzsche, Beyond Good and Evil (Gutenberg e-book @2009); section V.

Foreword for While You Diet
by **Arya M. Sharma, MD, PhD**

This is not simply a 'diet' book, nor just a resource about losing weight, but is a step-by-step look at how to improve your diet, your weight, your health, and your life.

Theodore Fenske, one of Canada's leading cardiologists and rehabilitation experts, takes his readers through the current science of healthy living. Himself a former vegetarian and marathoner, he has struggled with vascular disease and can speak from experience—both as a doctor and as a patient.

With ample references, illustrations, and a healthy shot of humour, Dr. Fenske discusses the concept of global risk—how risk factors for heart disease (like overweight, high blood pressure, high cholesterol) don't just add up but multiply to exponentially increase risk for heart disease and stroke.

Although there is much to say about healthy eating and exercise, the book also touches on genetic risk, molecular biology, and the complex sequence of events that lead to the formation of blockages in arteries, ultimately blocking the flow of blood to vital organs like the heart and brain.

These and other stories are woven around a 'day-in-the-life' that starts with a healthy breakfast and ends with the importance of sound sleep—yes, poor sleep is increasingly recognized as one of the 'root causes' of overeating and excess weight.

While the book is not written for those seeking a quick way to trim a few inches from their waistline, the book is certainly useful for anyone wishing to live healthier and prevent weight gain—should a few inches be lost on the way—all the better, but then again, health is not simply measured in inches or pounds.

Arya M. Sharma, MD/PhD
Professor of Medicine & Chair in Obesity Research and Management
University of Alberta,
Edmonton, Alberta, Canada

Table of Contents

Introduction

Things seemed strangely familiar as I looked up at the overhead compartments, stuffed to capacity with plastic-bagged medical supplies. It had been years since I had been in an ambulance. During my medical training I had spent many a weekend driving with the paramedics. I loved the thrill of the lights and sirens; the adrenalin rush of speeding through downtown traffic; the feeling of importance, being first on the accident scene; and the excitement of never knowing when the next call would come or what it would be. But I didn't feel any sense of thrill or excitement now. The ambulance attendants were noisily unpacking their equipment around me and I just felt bewildered. I looked at the Velcro straps tied across my chest, holding me to the stretcher. I had never tried out the ambulance gurney before, and now that I was strapped down to one, I wished the experience could've been indefinitely postponed. I could feel the paramedic tighten a tourniquet around my right forearm, and then the cool of the alcohol swab as he cleaned the back of my hand in preparation for an intravenous line. "Where are Tanya and the boys?" I wondered. I tried looking down beyond my feet to see outside, but the oxygen tubing was blocking my view out the back door of the ambulance. I tried shifting my weight to the side to get a peek.

"Now, try and keep still there, Partner," the ambulance

1

attendant advised, as I felt the sting of the needle in my hand. "Let me just tape this up, so we don't lose it."

I lifted my head up again. Now I could see the cloudless sunny sky that I had seen from my office earlier in the day; that Alberta blue that had called me out to "come and play." And I could also see the green leaves of the aspen trees fluttering in the lazy afternoon breeze. It was still summer and "Maybe one of our last warm days," I had said to my wife just an hour or so earlier. "I'm sick to the teeth with all this darn paperwork. I've just got to get out and get some fresh air. Why don't you bring the boys and meet me at the park?" I asked. And now, as I peered out of the ambulance's open back door, just above the tips of my shoes, I spied three frightened faces staring back at me in disbelief—my little boys, standing side by side, wide-eyed and speechless.

We had just arrived at the park no more than thirty minutes earlier. It all happened so quickly; it was during our first game of tag. My eldest son was *it,* and he was hot on my heels. "You can go anywhere on the play structure you want, Dad," he instructed me, "but the sand is out of bounds." Keeping ahead of him was no problem for me; after all, running was my thing—road races, 10K competitions, marathons. In fact, for the past six months I had been strictly following an intense training program to improve my marathon time. And all those hill repeats, track sprints and distance training sessions had paid off. I qualified for the Boston Marathon, and now, just ten days later, my legs were already recovered. I felt like Superman.

"Catch me if you can," I taunted my son, as I darted over the play structure, negotiating the rubber tires and rocking bridges faster than a speeding bullet. He enjoyed the challenge and I could hear him giggling behind me. And then my memory of events gets a little jumbled. There were the monkey bars overhead and I remember jumping for them—a simple leap that I'd done many times in the past. But for some reason, even though the bars were within easy reach, I didn't make contact. Instead, I crashed down into the sand below.

"You're *it*, Dad!" my son yelled triumphantly. "You touched the sand!" But when I started to get up and I looked over at him, his playful enthusiasm vanished and was replaced by a sudden look of terror, as if he'd just seen a ghost. "Mommy, Mommy!" he shrieked, as he turned to run. "Something's wrong with Daddy and he's scaring me with his face!" Little did I know at the time, but the left side of my mouth was paralyzed and drooping into a distorted snarl.

Now, as I peered out of the ambulance, all three of my sons had the same expression of fear and confusion on their faces. "Daddy's gonna be fine," I tried to say through the oxygen mask, but I had difficulty forming the words. I wanted to wave to them, to give them the thumbs-up sign, desperate to reassure them somehow, but I couldn't. I was tethered to the gurney. The paramedic was taping the intravenous line to my right hand and, for the life of me, I had no idea where my left arm was. I felt lost in a haze that was getting hazier, and as I tried to locate the left side of my body, my confusion

3

intensified. It was like waking up from an afternoon nap, when you don't know who you are, or where you are, and you just lie there perplexed and staring, with a drool bridge connecting your face to the pillow.

"Our E.T.A. is approximately seven minutes," I overheard the driver say into his radiophone as the ambulance door slammed shut, and any opportunity for "goodbyes" came to an abrupt end. "So long, my sweethearts," I whispered, as I laid my head back onto the stretcher and tears welled up in my eyes. The ambulance jostled me back and forth, as if to comfort me, while it rolled over the parking lot speed bumps, and made its way to the main road. The appointments and dates that had loomed so very important in my mind—my to-do lists, the research grant proposal, getting my journal article ready for publication, our new office expansion—all evaporated into insignificance. My only concern was for my family; their need for me and my need for them. Nothing else mattered.

"You'll need the stroke team," the driver added, as he ended his radio call and turned on the ambulance siren.

"Stroke team?! Why will they need the stroke team?" I wondered. My wife had used the word *stroke* as well when she had called the ambulance. "Was everybody going nuts?" I wondered. "Clearly this isn't a stroke, honey," I had explained to her (with my left arm dangling at my side) before she made the call. And you'd think I would know. After all, I was a cardiovascular specialist. For the past ten years, I'd been climbing the academic ladder in medicine, reaching Clinical

Professor in the Division of Cardiology at the University of Alberta, and Principal Teaching Physician at the Royal Alexandra Hospital. I wasn't a high-powered researcher or leading world authority by any means, but you don't need those kinds of credentials to competently recognize disease patterns and effectively manage sick patients. And managing patients is what I did best. With admitting privileges at a busy, tertiary-care hospital in downtown Edmonton, I was inundated every day by patients suffering from the effects of cardiovascular disease—chest pain, shortness of breath, stroke, collapse, sudden death. So doesn't it follow logically, then, that I would know best if I were suffering from a stroke? Not necessarily. Heart disease and stroke aren't constrained to our narrow ideas of logic. When a stroke comes knocking, confusion is part of the package, and I was a prime example of someone struggling with such confusion. Despite my paralyzed left side and the increasing difficulty I was having articulating my words, I stammered on, "Look, Tanya, I'm not having a stroke. It's just my funny bone is all. I must have banged it somehow on the monkey bars, and... well, as soon as the funny part wears off... I'll be fine. Let's just wait it out," I pleaded. "Don't call the ambulance. It'll just frighten the boys." But she would have none of it. With a determined look on her face, she sat me down, supported my back with one arm, and promptly dialed 9-1-1.

Within minutes, the ambulance lurched to a stop, marking my arrival at the University of Alberta Emergency Department. As the rear doors swung open, bright lights and noises flooded the cabin. There were serious faces, all looking down on me, worried. "The CT scanner is freed up. Take him there first," the triage nurse ordered, as I was bumped and wheeled into the emergency bay. A set of doors opened, and then another, followed by a long stretch of ceiling. "Funny thing," I thought to myself, as I was sped down the corridor. "I've never really noticed the ceiling before." Now, while being whisked to the CT scanner to have the cause of my symptoms determined, I had little choice but to either close my eyes or stare upwards as the ceiling tiles streamed past. No longer was I the doctor responding to a medical crisis; now, I was a patient in the throes of a medical crisis.

After the CT images were obtained, I was returned to the emergency room. The neurologist moved aside the curtain and introduced himself. "The CT scan confirmed that there's a blood clot in your right middle cerebral artery," he said calmly, and added, "It's caused a rather large stroke."

"Oh well, I guess that confirms that it's not my funny bone," I responded, to which the neurologist raised an eyebrow and looked even more worried. My denial up to that point about having a stroke wasn't entirely because of my hard-wired male bravado. I was suffering from what neurologists call *neglect*. The area of brain injury caused by my stroke had not only caused my face to droop and my left arm and leg to hang limp but also impaired my ability to recognize the left side of my body. But unlike the adage— what you don't know won't hurt you—this type of blissful ignorance can be fatal.

"There's still time for us to use thrombolytic therapy to dissolve the blood clot," the neurologist said in a hopeful tone. "And if we're going to limit the size of your stroke, we'll need to act quickly."

I nodded in agreement. Even in my confusion, I knew all about thrombolytic therapy ("thrombo" meaning "blood clot" and "lysis" meaning "break asunder"). During my early training years, I had the opportunity to give thrombolytic therapy to patients when it was first available for heart attack treatment. Back then, we wouldn't have dreamed of using such powerful clot-busting medication for someone suffering from a stroke; the risk of bleeding was felt to be far too great. In more recent times, however, it's been shown that thrombolytic medication can reduce the degree of brain injury caused by a stroke. If given within the first few hours of stroke onset (or preferably minutes), blood clot dissolving medicine can re-establish normal blood flow without the feared bleeding complications. Besides, if left untreated, a large stroke like the one I was experiencing could prove to be fatal or, perhaps worse, could leave victims severely and permanently disabled.

After I'd received the clot-buster medication, the neurology team re-examined my paralyzed limbs. "Still no reflexes; only grade one movement of the leg; and nothing with the arm," the resident reported to the neurologist, who then sat down beside me on the bed. He looked worried.

"The thrombolytic therapy hasn't worked as well as we'd hoped," the neurologist told me. "The reason is this," he went on. "The cause of your stroke ... is a bit unusual," he said slowly, as if trying to find the right words to break it to me gently. "We've discovered the problem and it's located in your neck. There's a dissection involving your right carotid artery," he explained. No further explanation was necessary for me; I knew exactly what he was talking about. The inner lining of one of my neck arteries had torn, allowing blood to clot on the inside of the vessel (fig. 0.1).

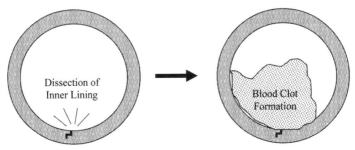

Fig. 0.1 Cross Section of a Dissected Blood Vessel

This type of vascular catastrophe, called an arterial dissection, isn't just confined to the neck arteries. Over the years, I've had to manage heart attack patients, who, for some undetermined reason, develop a tear within the wall of one of their heart arteries. It can be a real disaster. Over 80 percent of those unfortunate enough to suffer this type of vascular accident don't live to tell the tale.[1] The torn blood vessel causes a blood clot to form on its inside surface, which in turn can break off and drift downstream, obstructing blood flow where the vessel narrows, a process termed *embolization* ("em"-"bowl"-"eyes"-"aye"-"shun"). But not to worry; the likelihood of developing this type of vascular trouble is similar to being struck by lightning. By contrast, the vast majority of heart attacks and strokes result from long-term repeated injury to our blood vessels by a process known as atherosclerosis. The biological mechanisms underpinning heart attacks and strokes are very similar. Heart attacks occur when a vascular injury involves heart arteries and strokes occur when a vascular injury involves brain arteries. There are over 75,000 heart attacks and 25,000 strokes occurring in Canada each year.[2] In the United States, the numbers are even more staggering; nearly 2400 Americans die of vascular disease each day, which works out to an average of one death every thirty-seven seconds.[3] I've often quoted such grim statistics during my Powerpoint presentations at medical meetings and public awareness lectures, using pie charts and bar-graphs to illustrate the massive public health toll, and then adding, "as frightening as Mad Cow disease or West Nile virus may seem, heart disease and stroke are what's doing us in." Now, with my left arm and leg paralyzed and mouth drooped to the side, my own statistical opportunity hung in the balance.

"We need to try to repair your carotid artery with an angioplasty," the neurologist levelled with me ("angio" meaning "blood vessel" and "plasty" meaning "fix"). "It's possible that a well-positioned stent, or perhaps two, may be able to effectively mend the torn portion of the vessel and prevent further clot formation," he said. His eyes looked worried and his voice cracked as he explained the procedure, giving me the unsettling impression that it wasn't going to be routine. "Yes, of course. Do what you can. I'll be right here if you need me or have any questions," I joked, staring up at him from the hospital gurney.

I was immediately wheeled into what appeared to be a surgical suite, complete with bright, overhead lamps and a series of sterilized equipment trays surrounding a central operating table. "I'll need your pants off," said the nurse matter-of-factly, as I entered the room. "Oh, do behave!" I considered saying with an Austin Powers flare but didn't. Aside from the brief sting of local anaesthetic used to freeze the skin where the plastic catheter was inserted at my groin, the angioplasty procedure was painless. Since there are no nerves on the inside of our blood vessels, you don't feel the threading of the catheter, which, in my case, went from the insertion site at my groin, up the inside of my aorta (the largest blood vessel in the body), along my neck artery and into the smaller vascular branches of my brain. The injection of dye allowed the skilled physicians to locate the tear in my neck artery and position two metal stents, repairing the artery from the inside.

After the procedure was completed, I was taken up to the neurological intensive care unit for observation to recover from the day's excitement. The nurse in attendance asked me some routine questions to check my level of consciousness: "What's your name? Where are you? What day is it?" No problem there; I scored three for three. And then came the real test: the neurologist entered the room and asked me to squeeze his fingers with both of my hands. "Hey!" I said. "Will you look at that! Return of the prodigal limb. I can move my paralyzed arm and make a fist!" The timely treatments I received had successfully opened the blocked blood vessel in my neck and allowed me to enjoy a remarkable recovery from the stroke. On the third day, I rose again and walked out of the hospital, homeward bound.

Although innovative treatments have continued to improve the outcome of patients suffering from heart attacks and strokes, death and disability continue to remain a constant potential outcome. In fact, cardiovascular disease causes one-third of the deaths in Canada—more than any other illness—and represents the major burden of disease in our society.[4] Sure, we've had some success at reducing the mortality rate of heart attacks and strokes over the past number of decades, but the rising prevalence of diabetes, high blood pressure and obesity are undermining these medical gains. And, this is critical to note: to benefit from cutting-edge medical interventions as I did, you need to receive them promptly, and be mostly alive when you do so. Sadly, many people suffering from stroke present to the hospital far too late to be given disease-limiting therapies and nearly half of heart attack patients die before they even reach the emergency room. Better public education programs may help to improve survival statistics to some extent, but the only way that we're going to begin to get control of this rampant and snowballing disease called atherosclerosis is through intensified preventative efforts. Prevention of vascular disease is the thrust of this book, specifically for those struggling with excess body fat.

As we've been whiling away the years in front of our television sets and computer terminals, munching on taco chips and whatever else comes within arm's reach, we've laid down some extra padding—quite a bit of extra padding. So much extra, that over half of the North American population is currently considered overweight and nearly a third obese. And it's not just a North American issue; the rise in obesity is a worldwide phenomenon of pandemic proportions. It seems impossible to imagine, but obesity has now become the most prevalent nutritional disorder on the planet, outstripping under-nutrition and infectious diseases as the most significant cause of illness and death on the planet.[5] And most of this illness and death is secondary to cardiovascular disease. This is because those who are overweight or obese are at a significantly increased risk of having an early heart attack or stroke (fig. 0.2).[6] As a result, the only thing on the horizon that's looking slim these days is my dream for early retirement from my cardiology practice.[7]

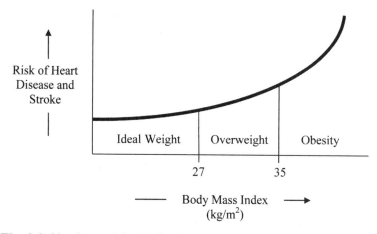

Fig. 0.2 Obesity and the Risk of Heart Disease and Stroke

Although some physicians tend to write off those who "have let themselves go," demanding that patients take personal responsibility for their health, I empathize with those who are battling with the bulge. We are all potential victims of the food industry's billion-dollar propaganda machine which relentlessly lures us to consume their products, our health and welfare be damned. Even though I've been a longstanding marathoner and committed vegetarian, I, too, have gained unwanted weight in the form of abdominal fat over the years and have been challenged to take more intentional and creative steps to keep trim. Weight control is a challenge for everyone; pounds can quietly sneak up and broadside our broadening sides, leaving us staring bewildered in front of the mirror, wondering where all those chins came from. Medics certainly don't help the situation any by handing out empty advice to their patients, like "You need to get in better shape" or "Try losing weight." Such vague and obvious suggestions do little more than embarrass and alienate people, and end up widening the gap between the available risk reduction strategies and the folks who are in most need of them.

Solutions to this extra-padding predicament abound. Or so it would seem when we scan the bookstore shelves and observe the sizeable number of rows given over to health books in general, and diet books in particular. But our dieting obsession has done little to diminish the pressing health issues of our day—namely the dramatic rise in diabetes and the continual onslaught of vascular disease—let alone rein in growing obesity rates. And it's no real surprise that adhering to dieting dogmas have failed to deliver their promised health benefits. Dieting isn't particularly simple, especially since we live in a highly automated world, surrounded by creature comforts, and inundated by tastebud-tantalizing, calorie-dense temptations. Most diets aren't particularly practical for regular living and many are too exorbitant for average incomes. While short-term attempts at any diet may bring some degree of weight reduction, long-term dietary adherence is rarely sustainable.-This tends to foster frustration and lead to yo-yo weight reductions rather than improved health and longevity. As well, dieting alone, as a solo health strategy, often fails to address the many footholds that cardiovascular disease can insidiously carve into our lives. Losing weight isn't the most important component of cardiovascular risk reduction and shouldn't be our solitary health goal. Besides, as Arnold Toynbee said, "The most likely way to reach a goal is to be aiming not at that goal itself, but at some more ambitious goal beyond it." In terms of weight reduction and dieting, this "more ambitious goal" at which we should aim is our cardiovascular health. Take heart, weight loss will surely follow as we take steady aim at this higher goal.

If you found this book in the diet section of the bookstore, I'm glad, since I'm convinced that the ideas developed in these chapters will be critical for dieters to consider as they wind their way along the path towards healthy weight loss and sustainable weight maintenance. But don't be misled; this is by no means simply a dieting book. While dieting concerns are addressed repeatedly throughout the book as inextricable components of our overall cardiovascular health, the discussions herein move past those of what to put in our mouths and what not to. As important as being overweight is as a risk factor for vascular disease, the ponderous paunch is but one cog in a complex wheel of factors that drive atherosclerosis and lead to heart attack and stroke (fig. 0.3).

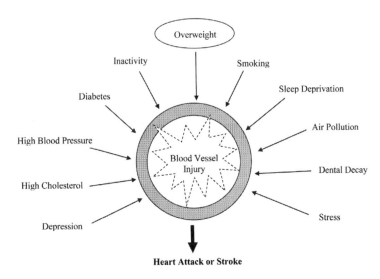

Fig. 0.3 Factors Leading to Blood Vessel Injury

The adage, "you are what you eat," is a blatant oversimplification of our biological makeup. It's possible to diet until the cows come home and not reduce the risk of cardiovascular disease in the least, and potentially even increase the risk. For health's sake, our food choices need to be considered within the context of a broader long-term approach to health, not as a standalone wham-bam-thank-you-ma'am quick-fix strategy. So, if you're looking for a book to help you shed those thirty pounds of belly fat before your daughter's wedding next month, put this one back on the shelf. I have no easy way, miracle solution, or short cuts to offer.

Nietzsche said, "He who has a *why* to live can bear with almost any *how*." While he probably wasn't referring to *why* cardiovascular disease occurs or *how* we can reduce the risk of having a heart attack or stroke, the truth of his statement can certainly be applied to preventative medicine; lifestyle changes are easier to adopt if they make sense. In the realm of diet and weight control, the gap between scientific evidence and popular opinion is a vast chasm, and it seems to be widening as we widen. My aim in this book is to bridge this gap with scientifically-grounded explanations that separate the dieting myths from the real deal. To move past the superficial treatment of popular health, I'll make use of illustrations that outline the key pathological mechanisms occurring within our blood vessels, where health and disease battle it out every minute of every day. And since few people are willing to wade through the dreary pages of a medical tome, I'll endeavour to keep things light by including stories from my medical practice, personal anecdotes, a smattering of historical tidbits and plenty of practical suggestions, which have grown out of my passion for educating my patients about cardiovascular risk reduction.

When faced with a frustrated patient in my clinic who says, "I just can't lose weight no matter what I do," I ask them to walk me through a typical day in terms of what they eat and what activities they do. Invariably, one or more red flags appear, indicating opportunities for improved weight loss success and improved heart health. So, in keeping with this approach, I've organized this book around a 24-hour time frame. Each chapter profiles a specific time of day, common to us all, presented in temporal sequence, from morning rise to evening rest. In keeping with Adelle

Davis' astute observation that, "every day you do one of two things: build health or produce disease in yourself," the chapters profile both how our cardiovascular system can be susceptible to disease and how its healthy function can be optimized during the particular time of day under discussion. The reason for using this "day in the life of approach" is to better connect what we know with what we do, and enhance the application of the material into our daily lives. To provide a more realistic forum for discussing practical risk reduction strategies, I'll introduce you to a composite patient of mine. Marion, who is a veteran dieter, and not only struggles with being overweight, but has numerous other risk factors for developing heart disease and stroke. As you join with us during her clinic visits, which open and close each chapter, I'll detail some sensible ways that can foster heart health, independent of weight loss, and discuss how both reducing the risk of vascular disease and reducing unwanted waist circumference can go hand in hand.

Our health is more of a journey than a destination point. So, regardless of the number of diets that you may have tried in the past, or have yet to try, vascular health can best be enhanced by taking a series of small intentional day-to-day steps in the same direction. As Teddy Roosevelt said, "We cannot do great deeds unless we are willing to do the small things that make up the sum of greatness." My hope is that the sum of "small things" suggested in this book will provide for you great success in building health and controlling weight, while you diet.

Chapter Notes

1. Baumgartner RW. Stroke prevention and treatment in patients with spontaneous carotid dissection. Acta Neurochir Suppl. 2008;103:47-50.

2. Svendsen A. The current status of cardiovascular disease in Canada— a call to action. Can J Cardiovasc Nurs. 2004;14(1):5-7.

3. American Heart Association Statistics Committee and Stroke Statistics Subcommittee. Heart disease and stroke statistics—2009 update. Circulation. 2009 Jan 27;119(3):480-6.

4. Statistics Canada. CANSIM.<http://cansim2.statcan.ca> (Version current at August 13, 2009).

5. Lau DC, Douketis JD, Morrison KM, Hramiak IM, Sharma AM, Ur E; Obesity Canada Clinical Practice Guidelines Expert Panel. 2006 Canadian clinical practice guidelines on the management and prevention of obesity in adults and children [summary].CMAJ. 2007 Apr 10;176(8):S1-13.

6. Adams KF, Schatzkin A, Harris TB, Kipnis V, Mouw T, Ballard-Barbash R, Hollenbeck A, Leitzmann MF. Overweight, obesity, and mortality in a large prospective cohort of persons 50 to 71 years old. N Engl J Med. 2006 Aug 24;355(8):763-78.

7. Flegal KM, Carroll MD, Ogden CL, et al. JAMA 2010;303(3).

Chapter 1
Wake-Up Call
Risks of Heart Disease and Stroke

Marion's Birthday Blues

"Here's the ECG for room seven," my nurse said, handing me the electrocardiogram just completed on my first patient, and added, "Be nice to her; it's her birthday today."

I scanned over the tracing. "Looks like a case of high blood pressure," I mused. "Wish me luck!" I said over my shoulder. Donning my stethoscope, I knocked lightly on the examination room door. As I entered the room I was greeted by a middle-aged woman sitting on the examination bed, barely covered by the blue, hospital-issue gown. She looked up over her Oxford spectacles and away from some tattered issue of *Good Housekeeping* that had been lying about the waiting room. "Rather stale reading, eh?" I opened, as I introduced myself with a handshake.

"That's alright," she smiled. "I'm always on the lookout for some new dieting ideas. There's one here called the Palaeozoic Diet which sounds promising—no gluten," she said, pointing to the article, with the hopeful tone of a gold panner spying some glitter.

"Well, hunting and gathering certainly kept cavemen

trim," I said with a smile. "But gluten or not, I'm not a big fan of diets," I added, as I sat down on the chair across from her. "Now, how is it that I can help you today?"

"Well, as you probably saw in my chart, my family doctor has some concerns about my risk of developing heart disease. I've had high blood pressure for a few years; I've been struggling with my weight; and my father died of a heart attack," she said matter-of-factly.

"Oh, I'm very sorry to hear that. How old was he?" I asked.

"He was fifty-three years old," she said quietly and then, after a pause, added, "the same age as me."

"Oh right, I almost forgot. My nurse told me that birthday salutations were in order," I said. "I hope you have more exciting plans for the rest of your day than getting a medical checkup," I added in an upbeat tone.

"Nothing special," she said gloomily. "I don't like to bring attention to my birthdays, especially this one. I'm the eldest of four siblings and, for the first time, I'm kind of worried about my health. My brother-in-law had some heart testing done while he was vacationing in Arizona last winter, including a CT scan of his heart arteries, and he was suggesting that I do the same. Is that available in Canada?" she asked anxiously.

"Perhaps not to the same extent as in the United States," I replied, "but, yes, we also have a variety of non-invasive imaging techniques that can help define the extent of heart artery disease in select cases. Is that what you'd like to have done?" I asked, trying to get some sense of her expectations. "Well, I don't want to wait until I'm having a heart attack... like my dad did," she said, with a hint of sarcasm in her voice.

"Certainly not," I agreed. "CT scanning has undergone significant development over the last number of years, but it's still a long way from Dr. McCoy's *Star Trek* "Tricorder," and there are some drawbacks. Viewing the heart arteries with CT imaging—called computed tomography angiography—requires a significant radiation exposure—the equivalent of 600 chest x-rays![8] Although the risk of developing cancer from such radiation exposure is still small, it does outweigh the benefits of doing CT angiography on everybody, willy-nilly. And even using the highest resolution scanners available, errors in analysis still occur, including the all-too-common false-positive results (that's where normal arteries are interpreted as being diseased, kind of like crying wolf when there's only a jackrabbit). And besides all this," I added, "the risk of having a heart attack or stroke doesn't just depend upon the mere presence of vascular plaques, but on how unstable the plaques are, and how prone they are to allow blood clots to form on their inner surfaces and disrupt blood flow."

Our blood vessel walls are under continual attack: stress, poor diets, sedentary living, and high blood pressure, air pollution— the list goes on and on. Vascular plaques develop as a response to this injury and they can potentially crack, or rupture, allowing blood to clot on the vessel surface and obstruct blood flow, similar to what happened to me when I had my stroke. Looking for plaques with imaging technologies may be well and good for patients with concerning symptoms, such as chest pain every time they walk on an incline. But the plaques we best identify with CT imaging aren't necessarily the types of vascular plaques that most often lead to trouble. Innocent-appearing plaques noted as only minor irregularities on the vessel surface go on to cause the majority of heart attacks.[9] The risk of vascular catastrophe relates to the degree of plaque vulnerability— how prone they are to rupture, form blood clots, and obstruct blood flow. Vulnerable plaques (the trouble-makers) have thin overlying fibrous caps and an increased amount of cholesterol within their walls. By contrast, stable plaques, the ones more likely to just sit like bumps on a log, tend to have thicker overlying fibrous caps and less cholesterol within their walls (fig. 1.1). Currently, we have no routine way of differentiating stable from unstable plaques, and we need to rely on what are termed *global risk factors* to best determine who is at risk for heart attacks and strokes.

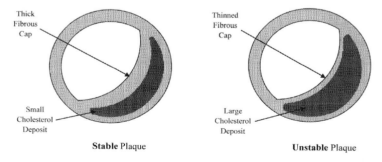

Fig. 1.1 Stable versus Unstable Vascular Plaques

Every Folk 'n Nation

Even though geographic, cultural and racial differences continue to divide our world, heart disease and stroke are indifferent to these divisions. There is impartiality to vascular disease that transcends the location of our home, our cultural heritage, and even our gender. When it comes to the risk of having a heart attack, there is no male or female, black or white, conservative or liberal, but rather, a potentially unstable vascular plaque in all. Heart attacks and strokes account for over a third of deaths each year, both at the farthest reaches of this planet and in our local communities. The risk of having a stroke or a heart attack (as over 70,000 Canadians do every year), depends upon the likelihood of having a blood clot obstructing the flow of blood inside a brain artery (stroke) or a heart artery (heart attack). Unlike my stroke, however, the vast majority of vascular accidents, heart attacks included, do not involve a traveling blood clot, or embolization. Rather, most heart attacks and strokes occur because of blood clots that form directly on the surface of an injured blood vessel. These clots don't necessarily journey downstream, they obstruct the vessel on-site.

What causes the injury to occur? A Canadian-based investigation team from McMaster University set out to answer that question, focusing their attention on the various modifiable factors that are known to accelerate vascular disease. Studying the patterns of heart disease in fifty-two countries from around the world, they identified nine factors that predispose a person to vascular injury. Since these same factors were operative in every country studied, they referred to them as *global risk factors*. They concluded that these nine factors could account for nearly 90 percent of all heart attacks worldwide (fig. 1.2).[10]

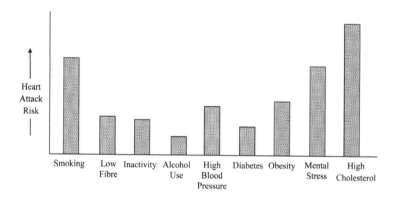

Heart Attack Risk

Smoking Low Fibre Inactivity Alcohol Use High Blood Pressure Diabetes Obesity Mental Stress High Cholesterol

Fig. 1.2 Global Risk Factors for Developing Cardiovascular Disease

Measuring Risk

The concept of risk factors isn't a particularly new one. In 1961, Dr. Thomas Royle Dawber noted a relationship between certain behaviours, like smoking cigarettes, for example, as well as certain medical conditions, like high blood pressure and diabetes, and the resultant likelihood of developing heart disease and stroke.[11] So, even before Ed Sullivan had recognized the Beatles, Dr. Dawber recognized that our lifestyle choices affect our health. He made a list of such associations and, checking it twice, he named them cardiovascular risk factors, and brought into being the discipline of preventative cardiology as we know it today. There are a variety of methods to calculate the risk of heart disease and stroke. The most popular risk calculator, and the one I use with patients in my clinic, is the modified Framingham Risk Score (fig. 1.3 for men and fig. 1.4 for women).[12] Despite the many novel, risk-prediction models out there, the Framingham Risk Score remains the gold standard for estimating cardiovascular risk and is fast and straightforward to use. All you need to do is plug in the numbers from six easily measured risk parameters, and you've got your ten year risk of heart disease; it's that simple. Two of the parameters—your age and your smoking status—can be filled in right now. The remaining four require a blood pressure check and a blood test for measuring your cholesterol levels (total cholesterol and HDL-cholesterol) and fasting blood sugar level. Points are accumulated according to your measurements. The higher the total point score, the higher your risk of having a heart attack within the next decade. Risk estimates less than 10 percent are considered low; 10-20 percent, intermediate; and estimates above 20 percent are considered high risk for heart disease and stroke.

Looking at the Framingham Risk Score parameters, age racks up the most points. Atherosclerosis is typically the result of repeated offence to our blood vessels ("Make it the usual dozen doughnuts with a double double to go, please"); so, it makes sense that the older you are and the longer you've been exposed to various vascular insults, the greater the accumulation of vascular injury and the higher the likelihood of getting stung with a heart attack or stroke.[13] But two points about aging and the risk of cardiovascular disease need to be emphasized.

POINTS	AGE	HDL-C	Total Cholesterol	SBP Not Treated	SBP Treated	Smoker	Diabetic
-2		>1.6		<120			
-1		1.3-1.6					
0	30-34	1.2-1.3	<4.1	120-129	<120	NO	NO
1		0.9-1.2	4.1-5.2	130-139			
2	35-39	<0.9	5.2-6.2	140-159	120-129		
3			6.2-7.2	160+	130-139		YES
4			>7.2		140-159	YES	
5	40-44				160+		
6							
7	45-49						
8	50-54						
9							
10	55-59						
11	60-64						
12							
13	65-69						
14	70-74						
15	75+						
Points Alloted							
TOTAL POINTS							

Points	Risk, %	Points	Risk, %	Points	Risk, %
-3 or less	<1	5	3.9	13	15.6
-2	1.1	6	4.7	14	18.4
-1	1.4	7	5.6	15	21.6
0	1.6	8	6.7	16	25.3
1	1.9	9	7.9	17	29.4
2	2.3	10	9.4	18+	>30
3	2.8	11	11.2		
4	3.3	12	13.3		

Fig. 1.3 Framingham Heart Study Risk Stratification for Men

POINTS	AGE	HDL-C mmol/L	Total Cholesterol	SBP Not Treated	SBP Treated	Smoker	Diabetic
-3				<120			
-2		>1.6					
-1		1.3-1.6			<120		
0	30-34	1.2-1.3	<4.1	120-129		NO	NO
1		0.9-1.2	4.1-5.2	130-139			
2	35-39	<0.9		140-149	120-129		
3			5.2-6.2		130-139	YES	
4	40-44		6.2-7.2	150-159			YES
5	45-49		>7.2	>160	140-149		
6					150-159		
7	50-54				>160		
8	55-59						
9	60-64						
10	65-69						
11	70-74						
12	75+						
Points Alloted							
TOTAL POINTS							

Points	Risk, %	Points	Risk, %	Points	Risk, %
-2 or less	<1	6	3.3	14	11.7
-1	1.0	7	3.9	15	13.7
0	1.2	8	4.5	16	15.9
1	1.5	9	5.3	17	18.51
2	1.7	10	6.3	18	21.5
3	2.0	11	7.3	19	24.8
4	2.4	12	8.6	20	27.5
5	2.8	13	10.0	21+	>30

Fig. 1.4 Framingham Heart Study Risk Stratification for Women

First, although the chance of having plaques hiding within the walls of our blood vessels increases as we age, heart disease and stroke are by no means limited to the elderly. The first patient that I ever managed with a heart attack was only twenty-seven years old. While his case was less typical and induced by cocaine, his case helped dismantle for me the fallacy that vascular disease is strictly an ailment of retirees. Half of all heart attacks and one-third of strokes occur in those under sixty-five years of age. Even children have been found with evidence of early disease within their blood vessel walls. A forerunner of the vascular plaque is called the fatty streak, a deposit of lipid in the vessel wall that can come and go over time. Autopsy studies from motor vehicle accident fatalities have shown fatty streaks in the heart arteries of children.[14] While the progression of atherosclerosis from fatty streaks to vascular plaque doesn't develop to any significant extent until after puberty in males and after menopause in females, their presence supports the contention that cardiovascular risk reduction is an important issue for everyone, regardless of age.[15]

Second, although everyone ages, not everyone does so at the same rate. Some people age slowly and gracefully, like the cinematic legend Janet Leigh, while others seem to take the fast lane to wizened grey and achieve that Ernest Borgnine look prematurely. Hard living certainly accelerates the aging process, and it's not just our outward appearances that take the hit. Well beyond the superficial reaches of Oil of Olay or Neutrogena Rejuvenator, the same aging process that is responsible for our crow's feet and etched foreheads, is also proceeding full-steam ahead at the level of our blood vessels. People with poorly-controlled blood pressure or diabetes, for example, and those with high levels of psychological stress or cholesterol, as well as those who smoke or lead a sedentary existence, all tend to have physiologically older blood vessels than those free from such trials and tribulations. Age notwithstanding, there is an extensive body of evidence that attests to our ability to significantly reduce the risk of developing heart disease and stroke by addressing these modifiable risk factors.[16]

No, we may not be able to turn back the hands of time and recapture that fresh, dewy glow of youth, but there is still time to slow down the aging of our blood vessels. Regardless of our present age, we can significantly reduce our risk of heart disease and stroke by agreeing to take some intentional steps down Health Avenue.

Family Ties

The global risk factors listed above, taken together or in some combination, may explain a great deal about why some people get knocked about by heart disease and stroke, while others live out their lives unscathed by vascular trouble. As well, the Framingham Risk Score can provide clinically useful information regarding who is at the greatest vascular risk. However, neither the list of global risk factors nor the Framingham Formula answer all the questions about the risk of heart disease and stroke: questions like why was George Burns able to defy all odds and crack one hundred years with a stogie in hand, while a poster boy for health, like me, barely scraped forty years without diving into vascular catastrophe? To flesh out the picture of risk assessment more fully, we need to consider how genetic inheritance plays out on our blood vessels.

My patient, Marion, had every right to be concerned about her family history. The fact that her father died at the age of fifty-five from a heart attack means that her risk of a similar fate is increased. While our genetic makeup may not be the dominant explanation for our longevity (or lack thereof), it's thought to account for about 25 percent of the variation observed in our lifespan. If your parents make it into their nineties, then your chances of doing the same are better than if they died of disease in their fifties. In particular, heart disease and stroke tend to run in families. Studies of twins have demonstrated that the more genetically similar we are, the more likely we will be susceptible to the same disease processes, heart disease and stroke included.[17] This is especially true for identical twins, defined as that situation where both babies originate from the same fertilized egg, or as my biology professor used to say, "Taking seriously what was poked at you in fun." When this two-for-one fertilization deal happens, both babies share exact copies of the DNA master plan. This means that they not only look the same on the outside (especially if forced to wear the matching sailor suits they got from Aunt Bea), but they look the same on the inside, as well. Since they're built from the same blueprint, it's not surprising that they share a similar predisposition to many diseases, including vascular disease. Studies have shown that if one identical twin develops vascular disease, the risk of a heart attack or stroke in the other twin is extraordinarily high: eight times higher for their identical brother, and fifteen times higher for their identical sister.[18]

The Framingham Offspring Study of 1971 also helped define the genetic influence of vascular disease.[19] Studying the outcome of over 2300 subjects, the investigators found that heart disease in first-degree relatives (Mom, Dad, or a sibling), significantly increased the risk of vascular disease in the other family members. This was especially true for family members who were on the younger side when they developed their disease; specifically, younger than fifty-five years of age for men and younger than sixty-five years of age for women. We term this condition of premature development of cardiovascular disease in the family, a positive family history. So, if one of your parents, brothers or sisters has established heart disease before they hit retirement, then your risk of cardiovascular disease is doubled.

Blue Genes

The study of medical genetics is an exciting one, with breakthroughs that seem to transpire by the minute. But it's not all late-breaking news. In fact, many of the principles that have given structure to our current understanding of genetic inheritance date back to the mid-1800s. The person considered the father of genetics conducted his experiments in the absence of modern technology and far from the spotlight of Science's who's who. When Canada was being put together as a Dominion, and America was being torn apart by civil war, an Augustinian Monk, by the name of Gregor Mendel, puttered in his garden and single-handedly shaped the conceptual foundation for genetic investigation by studying the secret life of peas. By carefully studying the stem length, seed shape, and flower color of over 28,000 pea plants, this holy scientist uncovered the patterns of inheritance which continue to serve as our contemporary framework for genetics. The discipline of genetics has evolved substantially since Mendel's backwoods beginnings. Fifty years after Watson and Crick's discovery of the double-helix, spiral-staircase structure of DNA (deoxyribonucleic acid), the Human Genome Project decoded this molecule of life, ordering no less than three billion building block chemicals to define its structure. Genetic technologies, such as cloning and gene therapy, are no longer merely material for science fiction writers to dream on, but are under active development and posed for clinical application. While our genetic advances have bounded forward, often outstripping our guiding ethical frameworks, one thing has become clear: the patterns of inheritance, particularly in reference to cardiovascular disease, are extremely complicated. Unlike the flower color or stem length of Mendel's pea plants, there isn't just one gene that codes for our vascular function, but untold thousands.

In addition, there's more at work in defining vascular health than just the DNA sequence of our genes or their number. Growing evidence has shown that our genes are sensitive to environmental cues. So it's not just the genetic code that's remarkable; it's how the code gets read as we interact with our surroundings. It's a bit like telling a joke. It's not just saying the words in a particular order, it's how the words are said, the emphasis, the use of dramatic pauses, the blank stare and raised eyebrow that separate a joke from getting polite chuckles versus one that gets an "Oh, my God, I think I peed myself!" kind of response. Likewise, our genetic risk for heart disease and stroke isn't solely dependent upon how our genes are strung together; it's also how the code gets played out and interacts with our surroundings. Our vascular health depends upon both the molecular sequence of our genetic code and how the code is used by our bodies.

The study of how our genes are managed by our cells is referred to as epigenetics. This field of research investigates the *how* and *why* of gene expression: how genes are unraveled and why certain sequences are read and acted upon, while others are packaged up and stored away. The role of epigenetics is to genes, as Brian Epstein was to the Beatles. Affectionately considered the "fifth Beatle," Epstein's tireless effort to secure recording contracts and promote the mop-top quartet with ever-larger playing venues was largely responsible for the group's early success. Management of any enterprise is critical to its optimal functioning, and genetic activity is no different. Recent studies have revealed that certain physical conditions activate the expression of some genes and deactivate the expression of others. This selection of which genes are "turned on" and which ones are "turned off" can have profound effects on our blood vessel health, since the expression of some genes are protective, while the expression of others can be harmful.[20] The dangerous state of uncontrolled high blood pressure, for example, can influence our DNA management system and silence the production of protective proteins, which are necessary to prevent vascular injury. The flip side is also true; engaging in regular exercise, for example, activates protective gene sequences that can help in vascular repair.[21] It's pretty heady stuff. Our gene storage logistics are enough to make IKEA furniture designers marvel and our cellular DNA strand compression system outshines anything that even Bill Gates could imagine. Fortunately, like the engine under the hood of your Dodge Viper, we don't have to understand the intricacies of how our genetic machinery works to improve our mileage. How we treat our bodies and what we expose ourselves to, play significant roles in how our genes are employed. The things we do or fail to do can have an important impact on our health by modifying how our genes are expressed. So, if your family history is dismal, take heart. Depending upon your day-to-day choices, you can carve out a much healthier path than your forebears did. Studies have shown that optimally treating risk factors can substantially lower the lifetime risk of heart disease and stroke, independent of family history (fig. 1.5).[22]

So, cheer up. There's no need to be blue about your genes.

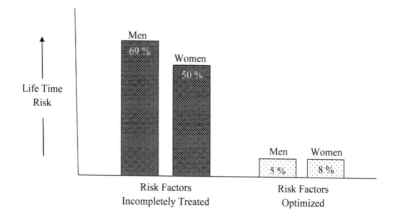

Fig. 1.5 Life-Time Risk of Cardiovascular Death

Is Marion's Number Up?

A knock came on the door and my nurse poked her head around the edge. "Special delivery," she sang with a smile, as she handed me Marion's most recent bloodwork.

"Good timing," I said and thanked her for the extra effort. "Let's calculate what your ten-year risk for heart disease is, shall we?" I asked Marion, as I thumbed through the results. "Yes, it looks like I've got all the information I need to make use of this risk calculator here... now let's see," I said, as I filled in her Framingham Risk Score Table (table 1.1).

Risk Parameter	Marion's Result	Marion's Number
Age	53-years old	7
HDL Cholesterol	0.92 mmol/L	1
Total Cholesterol	5.44 mmol/L	3
Treated Blood Pressure	148/92 mmHg	5
Smoking Status	No	0
Diabetes	No	0
Total Points		16
10-year Risk		15.9 %

Table 1.1 Marion's 10-Year Risk Score

"This gives you a number in the intermediate-risk range—a 15.9 percent chance of having a heart attack in the next decade. Unfortunately, however, this doesn't include your concerning family history. If we factor in that important piece of information, then your ten-year risk score doubles to over 30 percent. That plunks you into the high-risk range," I said to Marion.

Framingham Risk Score %	**X**	Positive Family History	**=**	10 year Cardiovascular Risk
15.9%		Multiply by 2		31.8%
(Intermediate Risk Score)				(High Risk Score)

"Well, that still doesn't sound too worrisome," Marion replied, optimistically.

"Yes, you're right. Your risk level could be worse—say

if you smoked, for example. But, let's not forget the lessons learned from the Titanic. Risk is not only dependent upon the probability of an event, like the so-called "unsinkable ship" colliding with an iceberg. Risk calculations are also dependent upon the final result if such an event were to occur, like having over 2,000 people's lives placed in sudden jeopardy as the ship made its way to the bottom of the North Atlantic. Since half of all heart attacks are fatal events, it's important to take steps to reduce your risks as much as possible," I explained.

"So, what should I do to reduce my risk?" she asked.

"Increasing the dosage of your blood pressure medicine would be a good start. It'll improve your risk score if we can maintain your systolic blood pressure below 130mmHg," I replied, as I handed her a prescription. "And regarding the testing your brother-in-law mentioned, I don't think CT images will change the focus of our risk-reduction management. If you have diseased arteries and we do nothing more than take pictures of them, it's a bit like disregarding the rising water level and proceeding to rearrange the deck chairs as the ship sinks. We need to pay attention to the proverbial vascular icebergs and do what we can to stabilize them. This will entail addressing a whole series of factors, including your elevated cholesterol, your diet, and your activity level. But for now, go and enjoy your birthday celebration!" I said with a teasing scold.

"Have my cake and eat it, too?" she asked sarcastically, as she gathered her purse to leave.

"By all means," I affirmed. "A birthday is no time to reproach yourself. Sackcloth and ashes can wait for another day. Go ahead," I encouraged, with tongue in cheek, "but perhaps, have just half a piece of cake and don't eat for two."

Chapter Summary
Wake-Up Call

- Unstable plaques lining the inner layer of our blood vessels can rupture and lead to blood clot formation, which can impair blood flow and cause heart attack and stroke
- CT imaging and angiography can estimate the degree of blood vessel narrowing by vascular plaques, but not their instability and likelihood of rupturing
- Heart attacks and strokes account for over a third of the deaths on the planet each year
- The risk factors that predispose to vascular plaque formation have been well-characterized and include smoking, diabetes, high blood pressure, elevated cholesterol, obesity, psychological stress, low fiber, and sedentary behaviour
- These risk factors are common to all people, male and female, in all ethnic groups and geographical settings

- Risk calculators, like the Framingham Risk Score, can help predict who is at the greatest risk for developing cardiovascular disease, and how lifestyle modifications can reduce our chances of heart disease and stroke
- Framingham Risk Scores above 20 percent are considered high risk for heart disease and stroke
- A positive family history of premature coronary artery disease doubles one's risk of heart attack and stroke
- Study of epigenetics has shown that we can modify how our genes are expressed and reduce our lifetime risk of heart disease by making healthy choices

Chapter Notes

8. Hausleiter J, Meyer T, Hermann F, Hadamitzky M, Krebs M, Gerber TC, McCollough C, Martinoff S, Kastrati A, Schömig A, Achenbach S. Estimated radiation dose associated with cardiac CT angiography. JAMA. 2009 Feb 4;301(5):500-7.

9. Schoenhagen P, Ziada KM, Kapadia SR, Crowe TD, Nissen SE, Tuzcu EM. Extent and direction of arterial remodelling in stable versus unstable coronary syndromes: an intravascular ultrasound study. Circulation 2000;101:598-603.

10. Yusuf S, Hawken S, Ounpuu S, Bautista L, Franzosi MG, Commerford P, Lang CC, Rumboldt Z, Onen CL, Lisheng L, Tanomsup S, Wangai P Jr, Razak F, Sharma AM, Anand SS; INTERHEART Study Investigators. Obesity and the risk of myocardial infarction in 27,000 participants from 52 countries: a case-control study. Lancet. 2005 Nov 5;366(9497):1640-9.

11. Kagan A, Dawber TR, Kannel WB, Revotskie N. The Framingham study: a prospective study of coronary heart disease. Fed Proc. 1962 Jul-Aug;21(4)Pt 2:52-7.

12. D'Agostino RB, Ramachandran SV, Pencina MJ, et al. General cardiovascular risk profile for use in primary care. The Framingham Heart Study. Circ 2008;117:743-53.

13. CV Risk Assessment: So Many Options, So Little Time. TK Fenske. Perspectives in Cardiology, November/December 2007; Vol 23 (10).

14. McGill HC Jr, McMahan CA, Herderick EE, Malcom GT, Tracy RE, Strong JP. Origin of atherosclerosis in childhood and adolescence. Am J Clin Nutr. 2000 Nov;72(5 Suppl):1307S-1315S.

15. Olson RE. Is it wise to restrict fat in the diets of children? J Am Diet Assoc. 2000 Jan;100(1):28-32.

16. Meir J. Stampfer, M.D., Frank B. Hu, M.D., JoAnn E. Manson, M.D., Eric B. Rimm, Sc.D., and Walter C. Willett, M. Primary Prevention of Coronary Heart Disease in Women through Diet and Lifestyle. N Engl J Med 2000; 343(1):16-22.

17. Scheuner MT. Genetic predisposition to coronary artery disease. Curr Opin Cardiol. 2001 Jul;16(4):251-60.

18. Marenberg ME, Risch N, Berkman LF, Floderus B, de Faire U. Genetic susceptibility to death from coronary heart disease in a study of twins. N Engl J Med. 1994 Apr 14;330(15):1041-6.

19. Lloyd-Jones DM, Nam BH, D'Agostino RB Sr, Levy D, Murabito JM, Wang TJ, Wilson PW, O'Donnell CJ. Parental cardiovascular disease as a risk factor for cardiovascular disease in middle-aged adults: a prospective study of parents and offspring. JAMA. 2004 May 12;291(18):2204-11.

20. Fraga MF, Ballestar E, Paz MF, Ropero S, Setien F, Ballestar ML, Heine-Suner D, Cigudosa JC, Urioste M, Benitez J,

Boix-Chornet M, Sanchez-Aguilera A, Ling C, Carlsson E, Poulsen P, Vaag A, Stephan Z, Spector TD, Wu YZ, Plass C, Esteller M. Epigenetic differences arise during the lifetime of monozygotic twins. Proc Natl Acad Sci USA 102: 10604–10609, 2005.

21. Margarita Teran-Garcia, Tuomo Rankinen, and Claude Bouchard. Genes, exercise, growth, and the sedentary, obese child. J Appl Physiol 105: 988-1001, 2008.

22. Lloyd-Jones, D. M. et al. Circulation 2006;113:791-798.

Chapter 2
Mending the Morning
Benefits of Breakfast

Marion's Morning Grind

"It's probably going to be high this morning," Marion predicted, as I wrapped the blood pressure sleeve around her arm. "I didn't leave enough time to get here and parking was difficult to find—you should really have reserved parking downstairs for your patients, you know!" she scolded me with a waving finger.

"No talking now," I said with a smile, inflating and then slowly releasing the cuff to get a measurement. "Yes, you're right. It is a little high," I said, as I returned the apparatus to the wall bracket and jotted down the reading.

"I told you so. I really had to bust my buns to make this appointment and now I'm a bit out of puff. No wonder my pressure's up!" she exclaimed.

"Negotiating through downtown traffic is no fun this time of day," I agreed, as I placed her chart on the desk and sat down. "But why so rushed? I thought you and your husband were planning to retire soon," I recalled, glancing back at my previous notes for confirmation.

"Best-laid plans of mice and men," she sighed. "Maybe in

a year or two, but for now we've got a houseful. Our eldest daughter and her two girls moved in with us. The divorce was pretty tough on them and Bill and I wanted to help out as best we could. So, now we're in the family way again, so to speak," she said with a smile. "And I need to keep working to make ends meet."

"I suppose that the last thing you needed this morning was to drive across town for a doctor's appointment," I said empathetically.

"Oh, I'm running behind every morning!" she exclaimed. "Between getting the girls up for school, making their lunches, keeping peace as they choose their clothes... and then there's feeding the dog and making sure we haven't forgotten anything before we leave. Even weekends are busy with their soccer games and dance lessons. I swear, it doesn't matter what day of the week it is; I'm running late the moment I get out of bed," she explained.

"Sounds like you're going off the rails on a crazy train," I remarked, and then wished I hadn't as Ozzy Osbourne's tune started playing in my head. "And where's your daughter in all this rushing about each morning?" I asked.

"She works at the airport and has to be out of the house by 6 a.m. So, we take care of the girls in the morning and do the taxi Mom stuff for her," Marion explained.

"What do you manage to feed your brood for breakfast?" I asked, wondering if the all-important morning meal might be getting lost in the shuffle.

"Breakfast?" she laughed, covering her mouth. "We have

no time for breakfast. The best I can do is grab a cup of coffee for myself and maybe a few yogurt tubes for the kids, and then we're gone," Marion confessed.

"Well, I can certainly relate to the 'hallowed be thy coffee,'" I said, nodding in agreement. "If I skip my cuppajoe, I get a splitting headache reminder; so, I, too, don't leave home without it. But, coffee alone isn't much of a breakfast of champions," I argued. "Not even enough time for a bowl of granola and fruit or a peanut-butter bread with some cheese before you hit the road?" I asked.

"Well, I'm not so hungry in the morning," Marion said. "And besides, I need to lose some weight," she added, pointing to her generous tummy and hips. "Skipping breakfast seems to be the easiest way for me to reduce my calories—although it doesn't seem to have helped much so far," she mused, now a little embarrassed. "But, I have a friend who not only skips breakfast, but often fasts into the day, and swears by it as a weight-loss method."

"Yes, there is a role for intermittent fasting in weight control," I agreed. "It can be an effective adjunct to losing weight, so long as it's paired with healthy eating habits and an exercise routine. But, that's not the same as skipping breakfast. Any diet that's worth following—and few of them seem to be—includes attention to a healthy breakfast meal. Even Dr. Phil's *Seven Day Plan* has a breakfast meal launching every one of his diet days. Breakfast is central to any successful weight-reduction plan. And, it makes sense: you wouldn't take your car out for a trip without filling the tank up first, right?" I asked rhetorically. "At the very least, our bodies need food for fuel to get us moving and help offset the stressors of the day.

"Here, let me give you a visual," I said, as I grabbed a pen and drew a circle within a circle on the back of her electrocardiogram. "Imagine that this is your blood vessel seen in cross-section (fig. 2.1). High blood pressure injures the inner lining of the wall, here," I said, drawing over the inner circle with my pen for emphasis. "But, so does stress— stress from running around with no time to even eat breakfast. There's no question that controlling your blood pressure is important to prevent heart disease, but it doesn't stop there. There's a large body of evidence that has clearly shown the association of regularly skipping breakfast with the risk of obesity, high blood pressure, and elevated cholesterol levels, as well as developing diabetes, and even the development of heart disease and stroke.[23] Slowing down to eat a regular breakfast will also go a long way in helping with both your weight control and your vascular health."

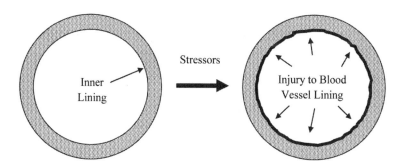

Fig. 2.1 Cross Section of Blood Vessel showing Lining Injury

47

Breakfast in America

Usually the first one up, my Grandma Sophie would shuffle into the kitchen in her slippers and housecoat, yawning and rubbing the sleep from her eyes. Her first task was seeing to the pets: letting the whining dog outside to find a bush and the nocturnal cat inside to sleep off the night's prowling. Then, after washing her hands, she would put the kettle on for tea and exclaim in her Irish lilt to anyone within ear's shot, "Ach aye, I'm famished. I haven't eaten since yesterday, ya know, and tomorrow will be the third day!" Banging of pots and saucepans would indicate that the morning meal preparation had begun. When she heard Grandpa starting to make his way down the creaky stairs, she would call out with tongue in cheek, "Is that you, Johnny, me love?" (His name was Harry, and her teasing always made him blush).

"It'll do rightly not to go playin' such silly games this early in the morn," he would retort, "at least not 'fore I've broke me fast."

For my grandparents, eating breakfast was a regular part of the morning routine. Just like getting dressed or putting a comb through their hair, breakfast was a priority for them. The morning meal was a time to gather as a family and celebrate the dawn of a new day. Filled with creamed eggs and soda-biscuit scones, and buttressed by Grandma's abundant affection, my mother and her siblings started out prepared to face whatever the day might bring. Theirs was an era when mealtimes were revered. Back in the 1930s, new immigrants like my grandparents didn't take breakfast lightly. Many fellow families of their acquaintance were challenged to get even one solid meal on the table, let alone three squares. So, with the long bread lines and crowded soup kitchens as a backdrop, they ate in gratitude for their good fortune.

Today, however, our ideas about mealtimes, in general, and breakfast, in particular, have shifted away from this grateful center. Our memories of the Great Depression are well faded and relegated to dusty textbooks or little disturbed photo albums in church basement archives. Abundant and relatively inexpensive food has now diminished the value we place on food as life-sustaining nourishment and our rushed pace has eroded the mealtime experience from precious to insignificant. Instead of beginning our day by sitting down to the breakfast table together as a family, we more commonly grab and gulp some powder drink mix and we're off. "We've come a long way, baby" in some respects—like being able to order a half-caf-decaf-skinny-mochaccino-latte and text messaging a vote for *American Idol's* top ten list while idling at a takeout window. But on the all-important breakfast front, most of us have lost valuable ground. Less than a third of North Americans fortify themselves with a proper breakfast regularly.[24] Many shamelessly reduce breakfast to some anemic meal replacement and delude themselves into thinking that the rich complexity of the day's most important meal has been adequately replaced by some highly-processed syrupy swallow. One in five North Americans scarfs down their first calories while driving their cars through cross-town traffic. Worse yet (as if anything could be much worse than careening down the highway, texting with one hand and drinking instant breakfast in the other), nearly 40 percent of North Americans make the morning dash from door to workplace without bothering to eat anything at all—and not because they're attending to an intermittent fasting regimen, either. They're just beaten by the clock and willing to forgo breakfast fortification to make up for lost time. Over the past fifty years, the once honourable meal of the morning has become the non-meal, commonly lost in the scramble and shuffle of chockablock schedules and teetering timetables.

Red Sky at Morning

It's an unfortunate series of events: our morning hustle and bustle coinciding with several physiological phenomena that, taken together, place significant stress on our blood vessel walls, and render them more susceptible to vascular calamity. Our naturally-occurring stress hormones, cortisol and adrenaline, follow a diurnal variation, which means they're more active during the day. The levels of these hormones are generally higher during the daytime, peaking in the morning hours, and fall off at night. So, as we're climbing out of bed rubbing the sleep from our eyes, our stress hormone levels are climbing, allowing us to face the fight of the day. Interestingly, this is the same time of day when our risk of having a heart attack or stroke is highest. On close inspection, the morning heart attack and stroke risk mirrors very closely the programmed pattern of stress hormone release (fig. 2.2). Coincidence? I think not.

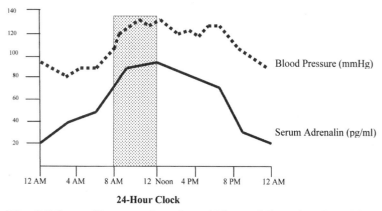

Fig. 2.2 Stress Hormone Levels and Time of Day showing rising stress hormones during the morning (grey box).

Population studies have indicated that morning time's a menace, showing a strong relationship between the time of day and heart attack occurrence. More heart attacks occur in the morning hours, between 6 a.m. and noon, than at any other time of the day.[25] In one landmark study, the records of nearly three thousand heart attack patients were reviewed and showed an alarming threefold increase in heart attack frequency in the morning hours, peaking around nine a.m. (9:30 in Newfoundland). According to their records, the safest time of the day, in terms of heart attack risk, was around eleven at night, "when all through the house / not a creature was stirring, not even a mouse." In patients with known heart artery disease, most angina attacks occur in the first hour of awakening in the morning, and 50 percent of all such attacks occur within the first six hours after awakening.[26] So, that feeling of indigestion during your wake-up shower may not be a Mylanta moment after all. If you've got morning chest pain, take warning, and get it checked out. The same is true stroke. Epidemiology studies have shown that more strokes occur during the morning hours between 10 a.m. and noon than at any other time.[27] In brief, the dawn can bring with it cardiovascular devastation.

Blood pressure elevation in the morning has been cited as the most plausible explanation for the temporal increase in both heart attacks and strokes. It's well-recognized that as we rise in the morning, our blood pressure follows suit and rises as well. The degree of morning blood pressure elevation is a strong predictor of stroke risk. It's been estimated that for every 10 mmHg increase in blood pressure during the morning hours, there is an associated 25 percent increase in the risk of having a stroke.[28] While this isn't so much of an issue if it occurs on occasion, it becomes a concern if it is repeated day in and day out. Considering that 20 percent of the North American population suffers from hypertension, blood pressure control is big business. Pharmaceutical companies are vying to cash in on the relationship between time of day and vascular events, expounding the virtues of their round-the-clock blood pressure controlling drugs. While anti-hypertensive medications represent a tremendous advance in reducing the risk of cardiovascular disease, we mustn't overlook the critical impact that our lifestyle choices can also have on blood pressure control. Studies have shown that when people take the time to eat a morning meal, their blood pressure decreases. This is important because elevated blood pressure exerts shear stress on the lining of our blood vessels, which over time can accelerate atherosclerotic plaque formation and lead to heart attack and stroke. So, countering this blood pressure rise by making breakfast a priority can help reduce blood vessel wall damage and, in turn, reduce cardiovascular disease progression.[29]

To help offset the havoc that stress hormones can play on our blood vessels, we need to make some repairs to our broken mornings. Rather than waking up in a flash and trying to make lightspeed to get to work, we would do well to recall the whimsical words of Simon and Garfunkel: "Slow down, you move too fast / you got to make the morning last." Bringing some organizational focus to the morning routine will set us onto a healthier path as we go "a-kicking down the cobblestones." Our priority in the morning should be to break the night's fast. It's the one time of the day when calorie consumption is not only safe but can be protective. Setting aside some time for nutritional calories in the morning not only enhances our all-important weight control efforts, but can provide some needed defense against vascular stress.

The Benefits of Breakfast

The importance of breakfast isn't just hearsay, but has been well-attested by scientific investigation, and unanimously endorsed by the medical community[30] Anita Renfroe got it right in her YouTube hit Momsense, when she included breakfast in her list of quintessential maternal imperatives. If anything, it should've been given extra attention in Renfroe's musical parody, so that it might stand out from the other caring commands. Sure, she said, "the experts tell us it's the most important meal of all." But, when the list is sung to the tune of Rossini's *William Tell Overture*, "Eat your breakfast" just blends in with the rest of the comical nagging. Much more than merely a motherhood statement, breakfast is a primetime, out-of-the-gate opportunity that we can leverage to build health and control weight. In addition to protecting our bodies from vascular stress, eating breakfast maintains energy balance, promotes metabolic health, and has the potential of providing our bodies with health-building nutrients.

When I review meal timing with my patients, I state loud and clear the importance of making time for breakfast. To avoid sounding like Mom nagging, I share with my patients some of the proven-effective reasons why the breakfast meal is so important. For ease of memory (and to give a nod to maternal sagacity), I've fit the key reasons into the acronym, WISDOM (Table 2.1). In this way, I can rattle them off to my patients in clinic as I underscore the importance of making breakfast part of their morning routine. On those hectic mornings when I'm also running behind, I can remind myself, so I don't fall into the too-rushed-to-eat trap, and succumb to skipping this all-important health opportunity.

W	Weight control
I	Improved nutrition
S	Stress reduction
D	Diabetes prevention
O	Optimize cholesterol
M	Mental efficiency

Table 2.1 The Wisdom of Breakfast

Breakfast gives the body a certain peace of mind, so to speak. Analogous to a consistent pre-authorized withdrawal plan for a charitable organization, having a regular breakfast provides the body with reliable energy input. Similar to how the charity can then focus on their mission at hand without having to overly worry about whether or not they'll be able to meet expenses, exposure to regular meals allows our bodies to maintain an energy balance without resorting to hunger pangs. This is particularly so for the morning meal, which breaks our nighttime fast. When we miss out on breakfast, we create an energy deficit that forces our bodies into playing catch-up for the rest of the day. This causes the level of the hunger hormone, ghrelin, to rise unchecked and produce no end of mischief.[31] In addition to stimulating our appetites with gnawing, grumbling ,and growling, ghrelin slows metabolism and decreases our body's ability to burn fat. Over time, the increased ghrelin activity promotes fat deposition, especially belly fat, and sends the brain carb-craving signals. So, as a result of habitually missing breakfast, we not only set ourselves up to overeat later in the day, but we become easy prey for sugary fare temptations like cinnamon buns, brownies, and butter tarts. However, if we start the day with a proper breakfast—complete with fiber, protein, and healthy fat—we provide our bodies with the requisite energy and rib-sticking fullness to get us through to lunch. This improved satiety stabilizes our metabolism, bolsters our appetite regulation, and helps prevent that midmorning weakness when ordering Timmies at the donut wall.[32]

Population studies of habitual breakfast skippers have given ample evidence as to the broad benefits of the morning meal. In one large cohort study, for example—spanning twenty-three years of follow-up, no less—the skippers didn't fare so well. They had an accelerated development of atherosclerosis and a significantly increased risk of dying from heart attack and stroke.[33] Researchers found that skipping breakfast is not only common in our society, but functions as a marker for unhealthy dietary patterns and lifestyle habits, including poorer physical activity patterns and impaired sleep. In addition to having more difficulty meeting healthy quotas of various nutrients of vitamins, minerals, and fiber, those who made a practice of skipping breakfast generally had increased cholesterol and triglyceride levels, and much more difficulty with blood sugar control.

This was particularly the case for those with diabetes, who experienced wide fluctuations in blood sugar levels and marked hyperglycemia after their lunch and dinner meals.[34] In brief, healthier people tended to make breakfast a priority, and those who gave it a miss ended up missing out.

While the morning meal has the potential to improve energy balance, help control appetite, and stabilize cholesterol and blood sugar levels, this is all merely just a *potential*. The only way of ensuring that our breakfast meal will live up to the lofty claims is by choosing healthy breakfast fare. Otherwise, the advantages of the morning meal are quickly lost, and may even work against us. For example, the type of fat ingested at breakfast can profoundly modify our cholesterol levels. If we eat too much saturated bacon fat or trans-fat laden danishes, we run the risk of increasing our "bad" low-density lipoprotein (LDL) cholesterol levels and reducing our protective high-density lipoprotein (HDL) "good cholesterol" levels. So, bacon-wrapped sausage lovers, beware! This upset in the yin-yang lipid balance of our bodies exposes our blood vessels to undo injury, and can lead to plaque development and vascular narrowing.[35]

Likewise, sugar and refined carbohydrates are also counter-productive to our health, particularly when consumed first thing in the morning. In fact, the worst thing we can do coming out of a fast is to eat sugary fare. This is because after a fast—even the relatively short eight-hour fast of overnight—our bodies are in a nutrient-ready position, primed to avidly absorb whatever we consume. As we've been moving through the various stages of sleep, our bodies have shifted from consuming and burning to a mend-and-repair mode. As such, our naturally-occurring levels of the anabolic "building" hormone (glucagon) rise, and the levels of our "breakdown" catabolic hormone (insulin) drop. When we awaken, then, our insulin levels are rock-bottom low and remain so until the first carbs start being absorbed, then slowly rise as needed. If we start the day with a sugar rush, we catch our insulin levels off-guard. This surprise attack causes our blood sugar levels to spike in a dramatic fashion, producing what's termed "postprandial hyperglycemia." Insulin levels follow suit, resulting in wide fluctuations in blood sugar levels, which cause insulin receptors to lose sensitivity. Over time, this leads to insulin resistance and sets the stage for developing diabetes. If, however, we choose a well-balanced healthy breakfast instead, we can prevent postprandial hyperglycemia and avoid this harmful glycemic variability.

For this reason, we need to give careful attention to both the timing and type of breakfast ingestion. This may mean avoiding certain breakfast options—even the popular ones—and intentionally making some alternative, and perhaps more creative, food choices (Table 2.2). Take instant porridge, for example. Although marketed as being low in cholesterol, this is but a smoke show to distract from the sugar content. One glance down the list of ingredients shows us sugar ranked in the first position. So, don't be fooled; low cholesterol may be nice, but sugar-packed is nasty. The same is true for sweetened fruit beverages. Sugar also leads the list of ingredients, followed by a series of unpronounceable constituents that read more like a chemistry experiment than food. Fortunately, there are alternatives for us to choose from. They may be more time-intensive and take some getting used to, but in the long run, they will set us up to reap the benefits of breakfast, and place us in a better position to build health and control weight.

Instead of this...	Try this...
Sweetened fruit Beverage	Natural fruit Juice (½ juice, ½ water)
Double double coffee	Coffee with skim milk & Splenda
Breakfast Cereal	Homemade Granola
Instant Porridge	Mixed Whole-Grain Porridge with Cinnamon
Pancakes or Waffles (gluten-free or not)	Oatmeal with Berries & Milk (no sugar)
Eggs Benedict	Egg White Vegie Omelet
Bacon & Eggs	Soft-boiled Egg with a slice of turkey & gouda
Scrambled Eggs	Cooked Egg Whites and Peanut Butter
Muffins & Pastries	Multi-Grain Toast with Peanut Butter & Sliced Banana
Scone with Jam	Peanut Butter & Apple Wedges
Toast & Margarine	Smoked Salmon & Cream Cheese on Open-Faced Bagel
Sweetened Non-fat Yogurt	Fresh Fruit/Berries with Plain Greek Yogurt
Granola Bar	Cheddar Cheese/Turkey Slice Roll-ups
Instant Breakfast Drink	Almond Milk Fruit Smoothie

Table 2.2 Healthy Breakfast Choices

Breakfast Bellyaching

There are many excuses my patients throw at me when I ask "why not" to eating breakfast—none of them very original, and certainly none that can counter the heaps of scientific data that support the regular inclusion of this most valuable meal into our morning routine. Here are some examples of what I get dished out in my clinic.

"I don't eat breakfast because I'm trying to lose weight."

Well, join the club! Weight control is on most North American's minds every single day. But, don't be deluded; the pounds aren't going to just melt away because you skipped breakfast. In fact, there are several reasons why your waistline may even increase. Missing breakfast typically translates into mid-morning hunger pangs, and that can cause us to make poor nutritional choices later in the day: opting for fatty, sugary treats over health-building fare. So, instead of settling for a skinny latte during the 10 a.m. coffee break, now you want a caramel macchiato with a honey cruller alongside. Don't fool yourself; the calories are going to come, and when they do, they'll likely come fast and furious, especially if you start your day hungry. You can choose to consume your healthful calories in a controlled fashion, as part of a nutritious breakfast, or you can scarf down empty calories helter-skelter, as you react to the emotional rollercoaster of the day.

So, rather than beating yourself up and complaining about how you can never lose any weight, take some action. Eating breakfast fires up the metabolic furnace and might even improve your ability to burn calories throughout the remainder of the day. Studies have consistently shown that eating a regular breakfast protects against the development of obesity and aids in achieving an ideal bodyweight.[36] By Contrast, skipping breakfast is a well-known marker of unhealthy dietary and lifestyle habits, total energy intake, and overall diet quality. The bottom line is that champions eat breakfast, ideally including rib-sticking whole, unprocessed foods and natural fats, and avoiding sugar and refined grains. I mean, why just fill the void at breakfast with empty calories and miss out on a prime occasion to build health? The key is to recognize breakfast as an opportunity to begin the day the healthy way.

"Pancakes and scrambled eggs aren't my thing. I don't like breakfast fare."

When you eat is as important as *what* you eat. If you don't like traditional breakfast choices, then break the breakfast rules. Healthy breakfast choices don't include flapjacks or bran muffins anyway. Open the fridge and get creative: there's nothing wrong with heating up last evening's dinner leftovers. The key is to avoid sugar and refined carbs and ensure, instead, you ingest something with a satiety factor. And, don't forget that eating breakfast increases the average intake of under-consumed nutrients, especially fiber-rich foods, like whole grains and fruits. For optimal functioning, the cells that line our blood vessels depend upon a sure and steady supply of anti-oxidants. Eating an orange, apple, or banana with breakfast—or, better yet, all three—helps to provide our cardiovascular system with much-needed nutrients. Making healthy breakfast choices has been shown to significantly improve our overall day's nutrition.[37] If you don't care for eating healthy food choices, then all the more reason to fill yourself up with them first thing in the morning, before your tastebuds have awoken and started demanding the wrong sorts of foods.

"Mornings are rushed as it is. I don't have enough time to eat breakfast."

Well, how long does it really take to cut up an apple and eat a bowl of granola? Sure, eggs benedict with hollandaise sauce can wait for the weekend (or, perhaps indefinitely, since we're concerned about all that fat and cholesterol consumption), but surely you can squeak out a few minutes for sustenance's sake. Skipping breakfast doesn't save time; it merely confirms that you're already out of time. A day that begins in a rush only gets more rushed as it unfolds. Mark Twain wrote, "Never put off until tomorrow what you can do the day after tomorrow." It is advice I gladly follow for such menial tasks as organizing the basement storage cupboards or weeding the dandelions from the front lawn. But, in the realm of countering morning stress, Twain's counsel misses the mark. Putting things off to tomorrow only overloads our tomorrows, and places undue stress on us when tomorrow becomes today. Procrastination invariably translates into morning chaos, where the breakfast meal is a common casualty.

To protect ourselves from this sort of stress, we need to build safeguards into the structure of our day, starting, of course, at the beginning of the day. Preparation and planning can bring needed calm into our mornings and make us less vulnerable to the adverse effects of stress on our blood vessels. The surest way to smooth out the morning routine is to iron out the wrinkles the night before. Lord Baden Powell's slogan "Be prepared" is worth considering. It's time-honoured advice that worked well for training untold numbers of scout troops for survival in the woods and will keep us on the right health path, as well. Making a few preparations the night before will save considerable time come dawn, particularly if you do happen to sleep through your alarm. It's quite a psychological boost to switch on the kitchen light in the morning and cast bleary eyes onto a breakfast table, already set, with blender and toaster on the counter, ready for a fruit and yogurt smoothie and a slice of peanut butter and banana toast. So, instead of doing without goodness, in less than five minutes, you can be munching on a balanced breakfast.

"I don't have much of an appetite in the morning. And besides, I get hungrier sooner if I eat breakfast."

We mustn't give hunger pangs a life of their own and allow them to control our eating schedule. Responding to every whim and fancy of our intestinal grumblings fosters overindulgence and leads to obesity. If you want to cultivate body awareness that will be of benefit, learn to sense satiety—and stop eating. Reducing our food consumption is far more beneficial than responding to our appetite's sweet little lies to consume more. A reduced morning appetite is often related to overeating during the previous evening. Rather than restricting calories in the morning and mindlessly consuming them at day's end, we would do well to heed Adelle Davis' advice to "Eat breakfast like a king, lunch like a prince, and dinner like a pauper." Front-loading our food consumption earlier in the day provides our bodies with the calories we need to work or play and renders our bodies more receptive for refueling the next morning.

The myth that once we start eating, we get hungrier soon afterwards, is only founded on the poor food choices of refined carbs. If all we choose to eat for breakfast are Twinkie-like options, then we can expect to feel hungry by mid-morning. When we eat simple carbohydrates, like breakfast bars and Count Chocula cereal, our blood sugar levels rise rapidly. Since our bodies are designed to maintain a steady metabolic state, skyrocketing sugar levels don't go unnoticed. This results in an immediate release of the hormone insulin, to bring sugar levels down to earth again, often too far down. This causes the midmorning feelings of hunger, which can lead to a snack attack. Over time, these up and down, yo-yoing blood sugar levels reduce our bodies' sensitivity to insulin and can increase our risk of developing diabetes. Fortunately, choosing protein and fiber-rich breakfast options, like egg-whites, whole-grain cereal, and fresh berries, can prevent blood sugar fluctuations and help protect us from developing diabetes.[38]

"Breakfast foods are too fatty. I'm trying to lower my cholesterol levels; so, I avoid eating breakfast."

True enough. Eating fried eggs with greasy bacon and a side order of lard-drenched hashbrowns or some poutine certainly makes for a considerable fat load. Such meal choices will undoubtedly increase cholesterol levels and the consumption of high-fat meals has been shown to impair the normal functioning of blood vessels and increase the risk of heart attack and stroke. But eating breakfast doesn't have to be synonymous with gorging on fatty foods. Studies have shown that fiber-rich breakfast choices can improve cholesterol levels: where our protective HDL-Cholesterol levels go up and our bad LDL-Cholesterol levels go down.[39] In the highly-processed food arena in which we live, it's often difficult to eat enough fiber over the course of the day. Breakfast is an ideal opportunity for filling up on this important nutrient that we shouldn't neglect. To boost the fiber factor and help optimize cholesterol levels in our house, we make our own granola and serve it alongside whatever the breakfast entree may be (Table 2.3). All the dry ingredients are first mixed together in a large bowl, and then the Canola oil is added and mixed in thoroughly. Add the liquid honey and mix. Place the mixture in a pan and bake at 275 degrees for one hour with frequent turning (every 15 minutes or so). When nicely browned, raisins and/or cranberries can be stirred in (1 cup in total).

Dry Ingredients	Quantity
Rolled Oats (large flake or a mixture of grains)	6 cups
Sunflower seeds	2/3 cup
Sesame seeds	2/3 cup
Coconut (unsweetened)	2/3 cup
Sliced almonds (raw)	2/3 cup
Whole almonds (raw)	2/3 cup
Whole pecans	2/3 cup
Cracked flax seed	2/3 cup
Wheat germ	1 cup
Skim milk powder (non-instant)	1/2 cup
Soy flour (low fat)	1/2 cup

Wet Ingredients	Quantity
Canola oil	2/3 cup
Liquid honey (heated in microwave)	1 cup

Table 2.3 Homemade Granola Recipe

"I need my sleep. Skipping breakfast lets me sleep in longer."

Benjamin Franklin had a sound retort for this slovenly excuse with his "early to bed, early to rise" advice. Going to bed twenty minutes earlier will provide far more restorative sleep than repeatedly hitting your snooze button with the declaration of dawn. Grasping for snooze snippets in the morning just takes the shine off the inevitable rise. "Up and at it then, and look lively," my dad would say, as he stripped my bed with me still in it, forcing me to retreat to the shower to find some means of warmth. Right up there with the hot shower and cuppa java, eating breakfast wakes up the body and prepares us for the day—and far better than what clean hair and caffeine can provide, a solid breakfast helps to counter fatigue, irritability, and that morning blah. What's more, breakfast gives us that essential mental edge to eke out our survival. Studies have shown that machinery and factory accidents are less frequent amongst those who take the time to eat breakfast before work.[40] And just ask school teachers for their opinion on the subject; they can spot the breakfast skippers within minutes of taking morning attendance. Children who don't eat breakfast are less alert, demonstrate lower levels of concentration, and are less efficient with their work, all supporting the idea that breakfast is, indeed, brain food. By contrast, students who eat breakfast score better on standardized achievement tests and struggle less with behavioural issues. It's no wonder that most inner-city schools provide breakfast and nutritional snacks to their impoverished students in so many North American cities.[41] Eating breakfast has been shown to improve memory and learning abilities in adults, as well. Since memory can't be expected to improve with aging, why not give your ol' noodle a fighting chance to keep up in our era of exponentially-increasing information by having a bit of breakfast in the morning?

A Stitch at Nine Saves Marion Time

"I wasn't always a big breakfast fan," I confessed to Marion. "Rush used to rule my roost. I'd run out the door with little more than a glass of orange juice on board and maybe a cold slice of pizza in hand. But, after my stroke, I stopped that sort of running around. It was as if a big pause button had been pressed during the most hectic season of my life and allowed me to make some healthy changes, including giving priority to breakfast. The evidence in favour of eating a regular breakfast is so compelling, for both improving heart health and weight control, that it can't be ignored," I said.

"Well, I'm not arguing that breakfast isn't healthy. I just don't know how to find the time for it," she complained.

"You don't have to prepare gourmet crepes with raspberry compote every morning," I assured Marion. "Even just a simple bowl of fruit and granola is a far cry from café solo.

I'm sure you've got time for at least that, especially if you add in a little strategic planning. As for me and my family, we made successful inroads into the morning scurry by getting our ducks in a row the night before," I explained.

"You eat breakfast at night?" Marion asked with a laugh.

"Not exactly eat it," I replied. "But, we've cleared away time in the morning for breakfast by doing some of the prep work the night before. In the evening, for example, I usually set the kitchen table, complete with napkins and cutlery, while the boys make their lunches and stack them in the fridge. After they brush their teeth, we have them put out the clothes they'll be wearing the next day; so, there's less time wasted futilely staring at the clothes closet bleary-eyed in the morning. Meanwhile, we set out what we need for breakfast. If pancakes are on the menu, my wife assembles the dry ingredients in a covered bowl, so they're ready for the addition of milk and eggs in the morning," I said.

"Sounds like pretty good teamwork," she agreed.

"I still get some flak from my teenagers now and again, but like the old adage, 'many hands make light work,' it's not particularly onerous for any one of us. Besides, children benefit from learning to take part around the house, even adult kids like your daughter. Bringing some organization to the morning, including getting breakfast on the table shouldn't be just your job. Trouble comes when we try to be too many things for too many people. Perhaps a dose of delegation might be in order for your household. Shall I write you a prescription?" I joked.

"If it means I don't have to up my blood pressure medications, I'm all for it," she replied.

"I can't make any promises about your anti-hypertensive medications; we'll have to keep a close eye on your blood pressure and adjust your meds accordingly. But, establishing a regular breakfast routine will certainly assist efforts to stave off vascular disease, and help you build health and control weight."

Chapter Summary
Mending the Morning

- Most heart attacks and strokes occur in the morning hours, secondary to stress hormone and blood pressure elevations
- For every 10 mmHg increase in blood pressure during the morning hours, there is an associated 25 percent increase in the risk of heart attack or stroke
- Habitual breakfast skippers have a significantly increased risk of dying from a heart attack or stroke
- Breakfast improves energy balance and appetite control and stabilizes cholesterol and blood sugar levels
- Front-loading our food consumption earlier in the day provides our bodies with needed calories for the day

- The key to a healthy breakfast is to avoid sugar and refined carbs and choose fares with a satiety factor, such as protein or healthy fats
- WISDOM acronym for the benefits of breakfast stands for: Weight control; Improved nutrition; Stress reduction; Diabetes prevention; Optimize cholesterol; Mental efficiency
- Fiber-rich breakfasts help to improve cholesterol profile, increasing good (HDL) cholesterol levels and decreasing bad (LDL) cholesterol
- Eating breakfast has been shown to improve memory and learning abilities
- Preparation and planning can bring needed calm into our mornings and make us less vulnerable to the adverse effects of stress on our blood vessels

Chapter Notes

23. Deshmukh-Taskar P. et al. The relationship of breakfast skipping and type of breakfast consumed with overweight/ obesity, abdominal obesity, other cardiometabolic risk factors and the metabolic syndrome in young adults. The National Health and Nutrition Examination Survey (NHANES): 1999-2006. Public Health Nutr 2013; 16: pp. 2073-2082

24. Timlin MT, Pereira MA. Breakfast frequency and quality in the etiology of adult obesity and chronic diseases. Nutr Rev 2007;65(6 Pt 1):268-81.

25. Muller JE, Stone PH, Turi ZG, Rutherford JD, Czeisler CA, Parker C, Poole WK, Passamani E, Roberts R, Robertson T,

Sobel BE, Willerson JT, Braunwald E. Circadian variation in the frequency of onset of acute myocardial infarction. N Engl J Med 1985;313:1315-22.

26. Willich SN, Kulig M, Muller-Nordhorn J. European Survey on Circadian Variation of Angina Pectoris (ESCVA) in Treated Patients. Herz 2004;29:665-672.

27. Manfredini R, Boari B, Smolensky MH, Salmi R, la Cecilia O, Maria Malagoni A, Haus E, Manfredini F. Circadian variation in stroke onset: identical temporal pattern in ischemic and hemorrhagic events. Chronobiol Int 2005;22(3):417-53.

28. Kario K, Pickering TG, Umeda Y, Hoshide S, Hoshide Y, Morinari M, Murata M, Kuroda T, Schwartz JE, Shimada K. Morning surge in blood pressure as a predictor of silent and clinical cerebrovascular disease in elderly hypertensives: a prospective study. Circulation 2003. 107(10):1401-6.

29. Ahuja K.D., Robertson I.K., and Ball M.J.: Acute effects of food on postprandial blood pressure and measures of arterial stiffness in healthy humans. Am J Clin Nutr 2009; 90: pp. 298-303.

30. St-Onge M.P., Ard J., Baskin M.L., et al: Meal timing and frequency: implications for cardiovascular disease prevention: a scientific statement from the American Heart Association. Circulation 2017; 135: pp. e96-e121.

31. Pradhan, S. et al. Ghrelin: much more than a hunger hormone. Curr Opin Clin Nutr Metab Care. 2013 Nov; 16(6): 619–624.

32. Astbury N.M., Taylor M.A., and Macdonald I.A.: Breakfast consumption affects appetite, energy intake, and the metabolic and endocrine responses to foods consumed later in the day in male habitual breakfast eaters. J Nutr 2011; 141: pp. 1381-1389

33. Rong, S. et al. Association of Skipping Breakfast With Cardiovascular and All-Cause Mortality. J Am Coll Cardiol. 2019 Apr 30;73(16):2025-2032.

34. Chang, CR et al. Restricting carbohydrates at breakfast is sufficient to reduce 24-hour exposure to postprandial hyperglycemia and improve glycemic variability. The American Journal of Clinical Nutrition, Volume 109, Issue 5, May 2019, Pages 1302–1309.

35. Uzhova I., Fuster V., Fernandez-Ortiz A., et al: The importance of breakfast in atherosclerosis disease: insights from the PESA study. J Am Coll Cardiol 2017; 70: pp. 1833-1842.

36. Elfhag K, Rossner S. Who succeeds in maintaining weight loss? A conceptual review of factors associated with weight loss maintenance and weight regain. Obes Rev 2005;6(1):67-85.

37. White WB. Importance of aggressive blood pressure lowering when it may matter most. Am J Cardiol 2007;100(3A):10J-16J.

38. Farshchi HR, Taylor MA, Macdonald IA. Deleterious effects of omitting breakfast on insulin sensitivity and fasting lipid profiles in healthy lean women. Am J Clin Nutr 2005;81(2):388-96.

39. Lipsky H, Gloger M, Frishman WH. Dietary fiber for reducing blood cholesterol. J Clin Pharmacol 1990;30(8):699-703.

40. Smith, AP. Stress, breakfast cereal consumption and cortisol. Nutr Neurosci 2002;5(2):141-4.

41. Morgan KJ, Zabik ME, Stampley GL. The role of breakfast in diet adequacy of the U.S. adult population. J Am Coll Nutr 1986;5(6):551-63.

Chapter 3
Coffee Break Caution
Concerns About Carbs

Marion's Toxic Waist

"Your nurse sure is thorough," Marion reported as I entered the consultation room. "After she did my ECG, she measured my weight, heart rate, blood pressure, and even put a tape measure around my middle. Since when do cardiologists care about measuring our middles?" Marion asked with a puzzled look.

"Ever since the epidemiological studies demonstrated that there's a direct relationship between waist circumference and vascular disease," I answered. "The greater the measurement, the greater the risk."

"Well, I told her to pull the measuring tape tighter," Marion laughed. "Oh, I don't know," she went on. "I watch what I eat and try to get out for walks when I can, but I still can't seem to lose weight... no matter what I do," she said in surrender.

"Part of the problem may be that you've entered middle age—you know, when your age starts to show around your middle," I said with a smirk, just as a light knock came on the exam room door, and my nurse's face peeked in.

"Her husband wants to join you. Is that okay?" she asked apologetically.

"The more the merrier," I replied, looking to Marion for her approval.

"Oh, sure," she nodded. "He's probably got my coffee."

Marion's husband was a large man and holding his winter jacket in one hand with two Tim Horton coffees balanced on a tray in the other, he filled the doorway as he entered.

"Looks like you've got a full load there," I said, introducing myself and helping him with his jacket.

"Every cup tells a story," he said with a chuckle, passing Marion her coffee, and then whispering to her, "I left the dutchies in the car for later."

I did the Bob Newhart nervous cough thing and turned to Marion. "But, that being said, calorie-dense food choices can certainly contribute to waist circumference. And in addition to padding the paunch, poor food choices can be toxic to our blood vessels. Sugary sweets, for example," I said, casting a raised eyebrow at Marion's husband, "can promote inflammation within the walls of our blood vessels. Vascular inflammation damages our blood vessels from the inside and accelerates atherosclerotic plaque formation, setting the stage for heart attack and stroke. But the good news is this: regardless of how much extra fat we may be carrying around, switching to healthier food items can decrease the inflammation process, with benefits that start immediately.[42] So, paying some closer attention to our diet, including giving some thought to our coffee break choices, can make a substantial difference to both our cardiovascular health and waist circumference."

The Central Role of Our Central Rolls

A tight waistband signifies trouble—and not just the need for a new pair of looser fitting jeans. Abdominal fat spells danger for our cardiovascular system.[43] The association between abdominal fat and heart disease isn't particularly late-breaking news. As early as 1947, French physician Dr. Jean Vague made note that his overweight patients were more likely to suffer from heart attacks than his less full-figured ones. But what is new is our understanding of the mechanism of how this occurs. From a heart perspective, not all fat collections are of equal concern. Excess padding over the rump, thighs, arms, or neck might reduce one's chances of making it into *People Magazine's* "Most Beautiful People" issue, but it won't affect your risk of developing heart disease nearly as much as abdominal fat. This is because fat cells aren't created equal. Depending on their size and location within our bodies, some are simply docile, energy storage sites, while others can be transformed into metabolically active tissue.

Abdominal fat is the transformed metabolically active type of fat. Referred to as visceral fat due to its location in and around our intestines or viscera, abdominal fat has a rich blood supply and a ready connection to our circulatory system. The hormones secreted by the transformed visceral fat cells are called adipokines (pronounced "add-Dippokines"), derived from the words adipose, or fat, and kinesis, or movement. These messenger proteins allow fat cells to "talk" to other cells, including circulating white blood cells. And this is no idle chit chat. Adipokines activate white blood cells, which then squeeze across the surface of our blood vessel lining and work their way into the layers of our blood vessel walls. Once inside the walls they become transformed into macrophages, Greek for "big eaters," and remove and digest any unwanted debris they come across. Despite their best intentions, these macrophages are like bulls in a china shop. As they carry out their appointed tasks, removing any rubbish they find within the walls of our blood vessels, they inadvertently leak digestive enzymes in the process. This is a real problem—worse than having your puppy leak on the living room carpet or your shower leak behind the backsplash. "What could be worse than a stained carpet or moldy tub enclosure?" you ask. When enzymes leak into the inner layers of our blood vessel walls, they eat them up and cause plaque formation. Over time, the leaked enzymes break down the support structures within the wall and can erode the fibrous cap that overlies the cholesterol-filled plaque and can make a stable plaque unstable (fig 3.1). If the fibrous cap gets too thin, it can rupture, allowing blood to flow directly into the inner sanctum of the vessel wall. This is like rolling out the red carpet for blood-clotting cells, called platelets ("plate"-"lets"), to gather together and form a clot on the vessel surface, which in turn can disrupt blood flow and lead to vascular catastrophe.[44] It's by way of vascular inflammation that abdominal obesity can accelerate vascular injury, leading to an increased risk of heart attack and stroke.

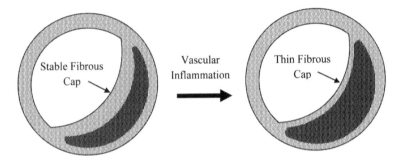

Fig. 3.1 Inflammation Makes Stable Plaques Unstable

Measuring Up

The risk of developing heart disease increases steadily with the increasing degree of abdominal girth. Recognizing this, medics are relying less on their stethoscopes to identify patients at higher risk for vascular disease, and more on their tape measures. Although waist circumference shouldn't be thought of as a fixed point of reference, thresholds have been established that correlate with heightened cardiovascular risk. For men, the waist circumference threshold is 94 cm or 37 inches, and for women, it's 80 cm or 32 inches.[45] If your midriff measures more than this, cholesterol-laden plaques hidden in your arteries are more likely to be harbouring inflammation, making them more prone to rupture and thereby nearly doubling your risk of heart attack.[46] Abnormal waist circumference values will vary somewhat depending on ethnic background, as well. Certain ethnic groups, particularly South and East Asian men, are even more sensitive to the inflammatory effects of abdominal adipose, and therefore the thresholds for concern are lowered to 90cm or 35 inches.[47] To see how you measure up, follow these instructions:

- Get yourself a cloth tape measure from a fabric store (the paper ones rip too easily and the metal ones don't bend well and are too cold against the skin).
- Bare your abdomen of any constricting clothing and stand with your feet shoulder-width apart.
- Loosely wrap the tape measure around your midriff, above the prominent bone at the sides of your waist called the iliac crest, at the level of your belly button (fig. 3.2). The tape measure shouldn't be pulled so tightly that it indents or marks the skin.
- Breathe easily and take the measurement to the nearest millimeter after you gently breathe out your air. (Sucking in your gut with a big breath is cheating).
- Record your number. If it's over 94 cm (37 inches) for men or 80 cm (32 inches) for women, you've got some work ahead of you to

turn off the fat-induced inflammatory response. If your number is under the threshold, it will be important to keep it there.

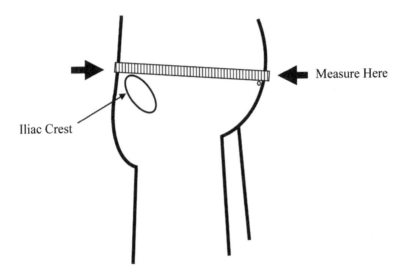

Fig. 3.2 Measuring Waist Circumference

Inflammation Constellation

In the 1980s, Dr. Gerald Reaven noticed a cluster of conditions—increased waist circumference, abnormal cholesterol, high blood pressure, and elevated blood sugar levels—all tending to occur more frequently in patients with cardiovascular disease. For want of a better term, he called this constellation of risk factors Syndrome X. Researchers have since shown that vascular inflammation can cause these metabolic abnormalities, and have therefore refined the name for the risk factor clustering as the metabolic syndrome. The mechanism is still being worked out, but this much is known: on the cellular level, too much energy in the form of blood glucose overwhelms our metabolic machinery. Excess blood glucose entering our cells results in the formation of highly reactive molecules known as free radicals and includes such nasties as peroxide, hydroxyl radical, and superoxide anion. Free radicals are like loose cannons and wreak havoc on the walls of our fragile blood vessels. By definition, free radicals possess an unpaired electron, which makes them highly reactive—chemistry-speak for "armed and dangerous." Free radicals not only damage cell membranes, proteins, and genes, but they also switch on our inflammatory machinery and send our blood vessels into a tizzy, initiating and perpetuating atherosclerosis, as well as a whole host of metabolic mischief.

When the inflammatory response gets fired up—like after you eat that dark chocolate mousse topped with whipped cream and caramel sauce—the liver responds by helping the white blood cells get rid of whatever perceived enemy is at large. The liver produces an array of proteins, called acute phase reactants that bind onto invading bacteria and viruses, providing the macrophages something to grab onto. These acute-phase reactants, also referred to as complement proteins, can be routinely measured in the blood. The best-known complement protein is the C-reactive protein or CRP. It was first identified during the Great Depression, around the same time that Sir Alexander Fleming discovered penicillin. Overshadowed by the success of the life-saving antibiotic, CRP got only second billing. However, in more recent times, it has been appreciated that elevated CRP levels— even minute elevations—can signify that inflammation is going on in our blood vessels, and studies have shown that high CRP levels predict heart disease. Not surprisingly, CRP levels have been shown to be higher in those with the metabolic syndrome.[48]

Fighting the Metabolic Syndrome

Five measurements comprise the metabolic syndrome: they include waist circumference, blood pressure, blood sugar, good cholesterol (HDL), and triglyceride levels. I've fashioned the parameters into the acronym FIGHT (table 3.1). This helps me keep them straight when I'm discussing the diagnosis with patients and underscores the fact that prevention of heart disease is an everyday battle.

Components	Diagnostic Criteria
Fat	Waist circumference > 94 cm (37 inches) for men > 80 cm (32 inches) for women
Increased BP	Blood pressure > 130/85mmHg
Glucose	Fasting blood glucose > 5.6 mmol/L
HDL	HDL < 1.03 for men and < 1.3 for women
Triglycerides	Triglyceride > 1.7mmol/L

Table 3.1 Metabolic Syndrome Diagnostic Criteria

To be diagnosed as having metabolic syndrome, you need to have a waist circumference measurement exceeding the defined threshold, plus at least two of the other five parameters in the abnormal range.[49] The metabolic syndrome, so defined, represents an emerging health burden for governments and health care providers across the continent. It's estimated that over 25 percent of the North American population meets the diagnostic criteria for the metabolic syndrome, and for the rapidly growing group of folks over sixty years of age, the estimate is closer to 40 percent.[50] Population studies have shown that people with metabolic syndrome have two to three times the risk of developing heart artery disease and stroke than the rest of the population.[51] What's more, this clinical clustering also predicts an increased likelihood of developing diabetes mellitus, a sobering sevenfold increased risk (fig. 3.3). And get this: if you're unfortunate enough to have four or more of the five metabolic syndrome factors, then your risk of developing diabetes shoots up to twenty-fourfold![52]

With odds like this, metabolic syndrome is certainly a condition worth fighting against.

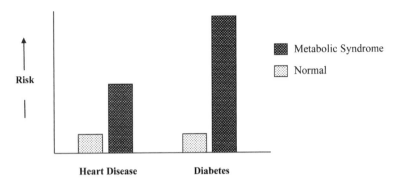

Fig. 3.3 Metabolic Syndrome Increases the Risk of Heart Disease and Diabetes

Coffee Break Broken

Our morning coffee break represents one of those times of the day when we can either build health in our blood vessels or add to our girth and produce vascular inflammation. Sadly, the choices that most of us make during our coffee breaks foster disease production. Although coffee can't really be considered a health drink, it's not the main culprit causing vascular mischief; rather, it's all those empty calories either added to or accompanying our morning mug that can bring harm to the walls of our blood vessels. While black coffee with no sugar and no cream is calorie-free, few choose this conservative option. Most of us opt for something more celebratory, like one of those specialty coffees on the overhead menu, and unfortunately, they're packed to the brim with calories (Table 3.2).

Specialty Coffee (20 ounce serving size)	Calorie Content
Tim Hortons Double Double	230
Dunkin' Donuts' Dunkaccino	460
Second Cup Caramel Corretto	490
Starbucks Caramel Mocha with whip cream	580
Starbucks Mocha Coconut Frappuccino	710
Starbucks Coconut Cream Frappuccino	870

Table 3.2 Calorie Content of Select Specialty Coffees

An average coffee-bar concoction has over 300 calories per serving, with some hitting over 800 calories in a single cuppa joe. For example, the Starbucks Venti Coconut Cream Frappucino, weighing in at 870 calories, is more of a milkshake than a coffee. If you then add in one or two baked goodies on the side—like Bill and Marion's Dutchies down in the car—you've really got yourself a waist-busting calorie overload. And that's just supposed to be a snack?! Considering that an average nutritious meal contains between 500 and 800 calories, it's easy to see how coffee break indulgences can quickly add some pretty big numbers onto the bathroom scale readout. If you want a coffee, then have a coffee, just not all those costly carbs on top. If you're concerned about either your ticker or your tummy, or both, choose the smallest serving size available (ask for a "short" at Starbucks), and skip the freshly baked brownie. As well, requesting skim milk instead of whole milk or cream, using sugar-free sweetener rather than allowing the Baristas to pump on the heavy syrups, going topless instead of adding the 'whip' (100 calories saved here, easy), and leaving the Timbits well enough alone, can all help limit excess calorie consumption during our morning coffee break.

But, the problem here is larger than simply the *number* of calories we consume; it's the *form* of the calories that's also important. Calories consumed in liquid form don't play by the same rules as do those consumed in solid food. This is because the mechanisms controlling hunger and thirst are quite different from each other. Our sense of thirst is triggered by water balance. When we take a drink and our body cells have reached a certain water threshold, our thirst is quenched. By contrast, our sense of hunger relates to the contents of our stomachs and the release of the hunger hormone, ghrelin. When our stomach and intestines get stretched from eating food, ghrelin levels drop, and our hunger pangs diminish. But liquids pass through our gastrointestinal tract too quickly to adequately stretch our stomach and turn off the release of the hunger hormone. As a result, our brain doesn't get the message that we've just drunk a meal's worth of calories, even if we have (and in the case of the Venti Coconut Cream Frappuccino choice, that's more than a meal). Since fluid calories don't suppress the hunger response, drinking calorie-dense beverages won't stop us from eating the same amount of food calories at mealtimes.

Beware the Ides of Starch

It's a curious thing, our coffee break culture. Every

morning at around half-past ten, they come—crowds of people—lining up in front of the donut shop at our hospital cafeteria. You'd think that Johnny Depp was there signing autographs, or Kim Kardashian was doing a photoshoot. It's a regular fast-food frenzy and heavy on the sugar. With all the consumption of chocolate croissants, cinnamon buns, maple dips, and Boston creams, perhaps we should rename our coffee break something more truly descriptive, like sugar-loading break, instead.

There are several reasons we gravitate towards sweet and comforting fare during our break time. First, we lead stressful lives. Our choice of coffee break goodies is, in part, a natural response to the hectic pace of our mornings. The psychological stress that permeates our workplaces causes the stress hormone, cortisol, to be liberally released. It's this stress-induced cortisol secretion that sets the idea of sugar plums dancing in our heads. Cortisol is centrally involved in energy metabolism during times of stress: mobilizing energy, so we can fight or fly, and then refueling energy afterwards, so we can fight another day. When it comes to refueling, fuel quantity trumps fuel quality every time. "I don't much mind the grade you use, just fill 'er up, Mac, and make it snappy," says the stress hormone. And what's the snappiest energy source? "Pass the sugar please," is cortisol's default response. This is partly why it's so darn hard for us to consume all those servings of fruits and vegetables that Health Canada recommends.[53] Even keeping to the daily recommended limit of 400 grams of carbs per 2000 kcal can be a challenge for many. This is because when we're stressed out, nothing seems to soothe frazzled nerves quite like sweets do.

Second, a missed meal is never forgotten: we either eat it now or we'll eat it later. If we miss breakfast, then the mid-morning break will naturally become transformed into a meal. Despite the casting of calories as sinful decadence by our diet-obsessed culture, we do need food energy in order to meet the mental and physical demands of the day. But we must guard against allowing our appetite to lead our food choices. If we wait until we're actually hungry, we set ourselves up for a dietary downfall. Those who skip breakfast are prone to cave into hunger pangs later in the day. When this occurs, it's common to consume too many calories and too many of the wrong types of calories, namely sugar. We need to anticipate this problem and ensure we make time for breakfast in order to protect ourselves from having a coffee break breakdown.

Third, a sugar fest begets a sugar fix. If we cave into the time demands of our culture and reduce our breakfast meal to a refined sugar moment of power bars, or crème puffs, or instant oatmeal, we can expect our blood sugar levels to plummet by midmorning. It's a vicious cycle of sugar craving that goes something like this: we eat a sweet treat packed full of refined sugar; our intestine says, "Go straight to the bloodstream, do not pass Go, and do not collect $200"; our blood sugar levels skyrocket upwards; the pancreas gets a panicked phone call—"It's happened again, I can't believe he ate the whole thing! Send some insulin! Do it now!"—

so, the insulin hormones put on their boots and race out the door; insulin levels rise to counteract the sugar coup; and insulin shoves the sugar molecules into whichever cells— muscle, liver or fat—may have a vacancy sign out front. But the scenario doesn't end with insulin efficiently getting the job done and us living happily ever after. Unfortunately, there is a time delay between the peak blood sugar level and the peak insulin level. That means that even after insulin has brought our blood sugar levels under control, more insulin is still being released into circulation (fig. 3.4). This causes our blood sugar levels to keep falling, triggering the release of the hunger hormone, ghrelin, which says, "Hey, I've got this hankering for something sugary sweet. Come on, indulge me." We respond by eating another sweet treat packed full of refined sugar and the cycle repeats itself.

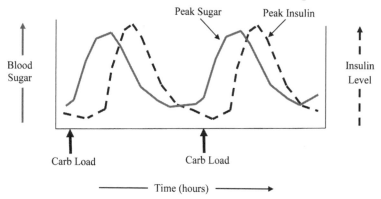

Figure 3.4 Peak Insulin Lags Behind Peak Blood Sugar

This sugar-craving cycle is painfully predictable and the results are brutal. Not only does the sugar craving cycle make us hungry all the time, but it also packs on the pounds. This is because whenever we consume more calories than our metabolic needs require, our body snaps into action and stores away the excess calories in the form of unwanted fat. What's more, blood sugar spikes place immediate stress on our insulin reserves and trigger a biochemical cascade, resulting in vascular injury. Over time, this increasing amount of abdominal fat, coupled with repeated sugar spikes, triggers inflammation within our blood vessel walls and increases our risk of developing heart disease and stroke. We need to wake up and smell the coffee… no sugar-coated donut, just the coffee.

The Low-Carb Camp

"Atkins shmatkins," said the server, as she generously ladled maple syrup onto my pancakes at our hospital's Klondike breakfast fundraiser. Her sneer summed up the current popular opinion about the onetime mega-popular diet. Doctor Atkins' diet once reigned supreme above all other popular weight-loss diets; but now the low-carb king has been derided, defrocked, and dismissed. Like most fad diets, the fall of the Atkins Diet was as dramatic as the rise. For millions of fervent followers across North America, it was quite a ride while it lasted. Despite the fact that less than 10 percent of daily calories were permitted to come from carbohydrate sources, dieters didn't seem to mind— at least, not when they first started the diet. There was so much newfound freedom at the smorgasbord table. Rather than complaining about having to give up potato chips and chocolate bars, dieters embraced the open season on meat and cheese. Atkins adherents could order their prime rib smothered in Béarnaise sauce, load up on the bacon and cheese omelettes, have a second bowl of that silky smooth avocado cream soup, and ask for triple cheese on their quadruple-patty burgers. The Atkins Diet was part of the dietary revolution that formed against the gotta-be-low-fat-to-be-healthy mantra of the 1970s and 1980s and was largely responsible for popularizing the low-carb craze that swept North America in the late 1990s. However, it wasn't long after we rang in the new millennium that the Atkins Diet began to lose favour. Even former zealots of the diet were starting to grumble and make excuses about why it wasn't working for them any longer. By 2005, two years after Dr. Robert Atkins' unfortunate and untimely death, his book sales dropped off, and demands for the Atkins' brand products fell steeply, forcing his nutritional company to file for bankruptcy.

Problems with the Atkins Diet abound: diarrhea, fatigue, and muscle cramps, to name but a few. For the cost-conscious, there was also the price tag to reckon with. Although sticking to an Atkins regimen was substantially cheaper than the pricier Jenny Craig or Nutrisystem diets, it was found to incur considerable costs nonetheless—80 percent more than what the average North American typically spends on food. Then there's the monotony: eating meatloaf and then more meatloaf, breakfast, lunch, and dinner. Dieters found the menu selection limited and tedious and began to covet their neighbour's croissants. From a scientific standpoint, the Atkins Diet was also found wanting. The Ketone Hypothesis, for example, theorized that if you forced your body to burn fat instead of glucose for its metabolic needs, you would lose weight by excreting ketone bodies in your urine. Well, that just doesn't hold water. And, from a medical standpoint, the diet is simply unsafe. Towering tomes of evidence caution about the cardiovascular dangers of consuming a diet high in trans and saturated fats, as well as the health benefits by their elimination.[54]

Even healthy young volunteers have been shown to immediately develop blood vessel dysfunction after consuming a single high-fat meal, let alone a continual barrage of fatty foods advocated by the Atkins' allies.[55]

While I was happy to see interest in this diet craze wane, we shouldn't completely dismiss Dr. Atkin's dietary approach to weight control. There are some important lessons to be learned from low-carb diets such as the increasingly popular keto diet. First and foremost on this list is that simple carbohydrates, and refined sugars in particular, are enemies of healthy eating and weight control. The success of the Atkins regimen had more to do with the sugary sweets that dieters were no longer eating, than with the fatty foods that they were eating in their stead. Just imagine, to keep with the program, disciplined Atkins followers had to say "no" to Tim Horton's donuts during the staff meeting, the double-chocolate cake at Aunt Jean's birthday party, and the bag of Fritos during *Days of our Lives*. Dr. Atkins proved that we'd been getting ourselves fat by overdoing it on the simple carbs. But since fat has long been regarded as the evil to avoid, most of us didn't notice that food manufacturers were adding increasing amounts of sugar calories to their low-fat products to make them taste better. We didn't realize just how much sugar we were eating until Dr. Atkins said, "stop." (Have you tasted how sweet McDonald's hamburger buns are?) Then, boom, pounds of unnecessary calories were removed from our daily intake, and weight loss followed. Secondly, not all fats are to be avoided. The demonization of fats by the medical community through the 70s and 80s not only set the stage for the carb craze but downplayed the benefits of a balanced portion of dietary fat. Natural occurring fats are beneficial.

While the contemporary Keto-dieters of the low-carb camp continue to argue that carbohydrate consumption is the central cause of our obesity epidemic and advocate for their near-elimination, common sense says "all things in moderation," and particularly so for complex carbohydrates. Many foods that contain carbohydrates, like fruits and vegetables, for instance, are an integral part of a healthy diet, with mountains of evidence to encourage their daily consumption. Although it's important not to demonize all carbohydrates, something needs to be done to counter our insatiable sugar cravings.

Smoothing Out the Sugar Peaks and Valleys

The speed with which carbohydrates are absorbed depends, in part, on the company they keep. Swallowing a solo spoonful of honey is like mainlining sugar; it hits the bloodstream moments after it gets past the lips. However, the absorption of simple carbohydrates, honey included, can be significantly slowed if paired with some kind of protein or fiber. It's a bit like the three-legged race at a church picnic. If you want to slow down Speedy Gonzalez, just buddy him with Slow Mo; now the chances of either crossing the finish line first have been greatly diminished. For a culinary example, consider the classic blueberry jam on toast. The jam is basically blue-colored sugar and the white bread isn't much more than sugar by the slice. They're both going to be absorbed into your bloodstream before you can say, "Pass the Frappuccino." However, spread on some peanut butter first (the all-natural kind, with no added sugar, just good old-fashioned ground-up peanuts), and the gastrointestinal absorption of the toast slows considerably, resulting in a much more manageable blood sugar rise.[56] Consider the table below for some further examples of slowing down carbohydrate absorption (Table 3.3). It's one way of reducing the wide fluctuations in sugar levels; so, you can have your snack and eat it, too.

Instead of This:	Try This:
Jam on WhTableite Toast	Peanut Butter and Banana on Whole-Grain Toast
Carmel Brownie	Cosmic Oatmeal Protein Cookie
Frosted Cinnamon Bun	Multigrain Raisin Toast with Cream Cheese and Cinnamon
Glazed Croissant	Banana Bread with a Slice of Cheddar
Granola bar	Cheddar Cheese/Turkey Slice Roll-Ups
Lemon Pudding	Protein Pudding
Chocolate Éclair	Quest Protein Bar

Table 3.3 Slowing Carbohydrate Absorption

To further minimize the skyrocketing sugar high, choose complex carbohydrates over refined offerings. Carbohydrate complexity refers to the *number* of sugar units strung together to make up the molecule. Some common simple carbohydrates include glucose (corn syrup), fructose (honey, fruit sugar), and galactose. They are called *monosaccharides* (the prefix *mono* means *single*; and *saccharide* is Greek for *sugar*). These single sugar units are already individually packaged and ready to be quickly absorbed from the gastrointestinal tract into the bloodstream. Other types of simple sugars are called *disaccharides*, or *double* sugar units, and include maltose (malt sugar in beer), lactose (milk sugar), and everybody's favourite, sucrose (cane sugar, white sugar, brown sugar, icing sugar, as well as coffee flavouring syrups, and maple syrup). Complex carbohydrates, or polysaccharides, are made up of long chains of simple sugars, called *polymers*, and include starch and glycogen. To get absorbed and used for work energy (or to be laid down as fat, as the case may be), the disaccharides and the polymers need to be broken down into their individual sugar molecules. It's simple enough work to cut the disaccharides in two, but there's a whole mess of bonds that need breaking before polysaccharides get past the intestinal bouncers and join the bloodstream party. In general, complex carbohydrates are going to take longer to be absorbed, and create less of a sugar peak in the bloodstream, than do the simpler varieties.

Dieticians use the term *Glycemic index*, often abbreviated to G.I., to rank carbohydrates according to their effect on blood sugar levels. Developed by Dr. David Jenkins, the glycemic index is a scale that specifies how quickly a given carbohydrate food gets absorbed into the bloodstream by comparison to the reference of fifty grams of oral glucose. Carbohydrates with a low glycemic index (less than fifty-five), are absorbed more slowly and result in less of a blood sugar elevation than their counterparts with higher indices. For example, a snack of white bread and jelly with a glycemic index of eighty will result in a blood sugar peak that is twice as high as a whole-grain bread and peanut butter with a glycemic index of forty. This is important, since the faster a carbohydrate gets dismantled into simple sugar, the higher the resultant blood sugar peak; and the higher the peak, the more the stress on our blood vessels and the more fat on our abdomens. Studies have shown that diets rich in high-glycemic-index, low-fiber foods increase the risk of both cardiovascular disease and diabetes.[57] So, when you're looking for carbohydrates as part of your regularly planned meals, it's best to choose complex carbohydrates with a low glycemic index (table 3.4).

	Glycemic Index Below 55 (Good)	Glycemic Index Above 55 (Not As Good)
Fruit	Pears, peaches, plums, apples, grapefruit	Pineapple, watermelon, apricots, raisins, dates
Vegetables	Asparagus, broccoli, chickpeas, yams	Baked potatoes, parsnips, broad beans
Grains	Whole wheat spaghetti, multigrain bread, parboiled wild rice, non-instant porridge, granola	White bread and buns, white rice, white pasta, crackers, pastries, croissants, donuts, cakes, tarts, muffins...
Snacks	Roasted almonds	Jelly beans, corn chips, pretzels

Table 3.4 Carbohydrates According to Glycemic Index

Rather than memorizing some dreary dietary list of less-desirable simple carbohydrates versus more-preferable complex carbohydrates, consider it this way instead: processed foods contain simple, refined sugars and are to be avoided; natural foods contain more complex carbohydrates and are more preferable. One exception would be fruits like pineapple or watermelon, which happen to be packed full of fructose, the fruit sugar. However, despite high glycemic indices, fruits still outshine processed carbs because they have fewer calories, higher water and fiber content, and they are excellent sources of vitamins and minerals. So, to avoid the worst carbs, simply avoid processed treats, including donuts, tarts, buns, and crackers, and go for the fruit basket instead. In the confusing world of dieting, one thing is certain: if Mother Nature made it, it's going to be a lot healthier than something from Aunt Jemima.

Waist Not Want Not

"I've got so much weight to lose, it's overwhelming," Marion confessed. "And at the rate I'm going, there's no way that I can lose it all. I know; I've tried all the diets, and they might help me initially, but I can never keep the weight off," she said.

"Who said anything about losing *all the weight*? You don't have to look like Twiggy to improve your heart health, you know," I countered.

"Yeah, well, I look more like *three* Twiggys," she sighed.

"And I'm probably a four-plus," her husband, Bill, piped in with a chuckle.

"Weigh scales aren't the only measure of health," I said to them both. "Besides, we're not trying to launch a modeling career here. The key issue for each of us is maintaining the health of our blood vessels so we don't die of a premature heart attack or stroke. Sure, it's important that you stop gaining weight—that's the first goal; and then tip the scale in the right direction—that's the second. But, you don't have to be reduced to skin and bones to turn down the inflammation going on in your blood vessel walls. Studies have shown that a small weight loss of only 5 to 10 percent can substantially reduce the risk of cardiovascular disease.[58] That means taking off, let's say, ten or fifteen pounds to start with. Not so impossible, eh?" I asked.

"I suppose not," Marion agreed. "But do you mean to tell me that if I lose just ten pounds that I'm no longer at risk for heart disease?" she asked, scrunching up her face in disbelief.

"Wouldn't that be a wonderful life," I answered. "Not even the lean, mean Olympians like Michael Phelps can boast a cardiovascular risk of nil," I countered. "The risk of developing heart disease and stroke isn't an all or none thing. It's more like your mortgage payment; it's always there, but with a little planning, it doesn't have to break you. While the risk of having a heart attack or stroke can't be eliminated completely, we can still make some significant headway on improving both the quantity and quality of our lives."

"So, where do you suggest that we start?" she asked.

"How about starting with today's coffee break," I smiled. "I've got an apple and a banana waiting for me at my break time. So, when you get down to the car, why don't you lose the Dutchies and choose a healthy snack like mine, instead."

"Throw out our donuts?!" Bill questioned, sounding alarmed.

"Hey, they're better in the wastebasket now," I replied, motioning to the garbage container, "than on the waist, forever," I added, patting my sides. "Besides, there's no time like the present to break that vicious sugar cycle, and the surest way to do it is by going cold turkey. Smokers know this all too well. Nicotine patches, gum, mood stabilizers, hypnosis, acupuncture, meditation may all help, but to successfully quit smoking, they finally have to butt out."

"Are you saying no carbs?! That sounds a lot like the Atkins Diet. I tried that one, too," Marion shared.

"Well, I'm not advocating a complete embargo on carbohydrates. There's just too much nutritionally sound food under that broad umbrella to leave complex carbohydrates out of our diets. How about taking a sugar holiday? A full two weeks with no refined carbs would force a healthy rethink about meals and snacks, and might just get you on the right path to start breaking some of those sugar addiction bonds. Why, even just a one day sugar Sabbath would be a step in the right direction. And, who knows, maybe in time, you'll end up preferring an apple over an apple fritter."

"I suppose we could think about it," Marion said unconvincingly. "But it's going to be so hard to give up our coffee break snacks... it's something we've done forever."

"Yes, new tricks can be difficult to learn," I agreed. Pulling out a copy of my wife's Cranberry Banana Bread recipe from the accordion file on my desk (Fig. 3.5), I countered, "How about baking a healthy snack, instead? My wife uses this recipe. It's loaded with tart cranberries, sweet chocolate chips and lots of nuts. She substitutes apple sauce for half the amount of oil and reduces the sugar content substantially, as well. Our boys love it, and with a piece of cheese, it makes a much better coffee companion than anything Timmies has to offer. Bon Appétit!"

DRY INGREDIENTS:
1 ½ cups whole wheat flour
2 cups all-purpose flour
2 tsp baking soda
1 ½ cups sugar
1 tsp salt
1 cup frozen or fresh cranberries (not dried)
¾ cup chocolate chips
1 ½ cups roughly chopped pecans
WET INGREDIENTS:
4 large eggs
2 cups mashed ripe bananas (4 large bananas)
½ cup cooking oil
½ cup unsweetened applesauce *
¾ cup buttermilk, or yoghurt and milk mixed together
2 tsp vanilla

Substitute applesauce for half the oil in most muffin/loaf recipes. The snack-sized containers that kids take for lunches are often a ½ cup, and they are easy to keep available in your pantry.

METHOD:
1. Grease & flour two 5 X 9" loafpans. Preheat oven to 325°
2. In separate bowls, mix the wet and dry ingredients.
3. Pour the wet mixture into the dry and stir until just moistened.
4. Divide into the loafpans and bake for about 1 hour and 10 minutes, but start to check for doneness after 1 hour or so.*(To make muffins, bake for 30-40 minutes instead.)*
5. Cool in the pans for 10 minutes, and then turn out onto cooling racks.
6. When cool, wrap tightly in plastic. Store for 2-3 days in the fridge, or freeze for later use

Fig. 3.5 Cranberry Banana Bread Recipe

Chapter Summary
Coffee Break Caution

- Abdominal fat is metabolically active and associated with vascular inflammation
- Abdominal fat can be estimated by measuring waist circumference
- Waist circumference thresholds of > 94 cm (37 inches) for men and > 80 cm (32 inches) for women are associated with an increased heart disease risk
- The metabolic syndrome comprises a cluster of conditions that produce blood vessel inflammation and heighten the risk of developing diabetes and heart disease
- The acronym FIGHT represents the five elements of the metabolic syndrome and stands for Fat, Increased blood pressure, Glucose elevation, HDL reduction, and Triglyceride elevation
- Reducing simple carbohydrate consumption can help reduce the risk of developing metabolic syndrome
- Avoid blood sugar peaks by either avoiding simple carbs or pairing them with protein or fiber to slow absorption time
- Many high-calorie coffee beverages contain sugar

and should be avoided
- Coffee breaks need not be a sugar fest
- Healthier coffee break snack options have a satiety factor, like protein or fat
- Carbohydrates with a glycemic index of less than fifty-five are absorbed more slowly and are less likely to lead to insulin resistance
- Snacks can be made healthier by reducing sugar content and by using fat substitutes, like applesauce

Chapter Notes

42. O'Keefe JH, Neil MD, Gheewala MS, O'Keefe JO. Dietary strategies for improving post-prandial glucose, lipids, inflammation, and cardiovascular health. J Am Coll Cardiol 2008;51:249-55.

43. Abdominal fat and cardiovascular disease risk (p. 142) Després JP, Lemieux I, Bergeron J, Pibarot P, Mathieu P, Larose E, Rodés-Cabau J, Bertrand OF, Poirier P. Abdominal obesity and the metabolic syndrome: contribution to global cardiometabolic risk. Arterioscler Thromb Vasc Biol. 2008 Jun;28(6):1039-49.

44. Insull W. The Pathology of Atherosclerosis: Plaque Development and Plaque Responses to Medical Treatment. Am J Med 2009;122(Suppl1):S3-S14.

45. Alberti KG, Zimmet P, Shaw J. Metabolic syndrome—a new world-wide definition. A Consensus Statement from the International Diabetes Federation. Diabet Med 2006;23(5):469-480.

46. Atherosclerosis Risk in Communities Study. Am J Cardiol

2004;94 (10):1249-54.

47. Jafar TH, Chaturvedi N, Pappas G. Prevalence of overweight and obesity and their association with hypertension and diabetes mellitus in an Indo-Asian population. CMAJ 2006;175(9):1071-1077.

48. Florez H, Castillo-Florez S, Mendez A, Casanova-Romero P, Larreal-Urdaneta C, Lee D, Goldberg R.C-reactive protein is elevated in obese patients with the metabolic syndrome. Diabetes Res Clin Pract. 2006 Jan;71(1):92-100.

49. Alberti KG, Zimmet P, Shaw J; IDF Epidemiology Task Force Consensus Group. The Metabolic Syndrome - a new worldwide definition. Lancet 2005;366:1059-62.

50. Lutsey PL, Steffen LM, Stevens J. Dietary intake and the development of the metabolic syndrome: the Atherosclerosis Risk in Communities study. Circulation. 2008 Feb 12;117(6):754-61.

51. Després JP, Lemieux I, Bergeron J, Pibarot P, Mathieu P, Larose E, Rodés-Cabau J, Bertrand OF, Poirier P. Abdominal obesity and the metabolic syndrome: contribution to global cardiometabolic risk. Arterioscler Thromb Vasc Biol. 2008 Jun;28(6):1039-49.

52. Sattar N, Gaw A, Scherbakova O, Ford I, O'Reilly DS, Haffner SM, Isles C, Macfarlane PW, Packard CJ, Cobbe SM, Shepherd J. Metabolic syndrome with and without C-reactive protein as a predictor of coronary heart disease and diabetes in the West of Scotland Coronary Prevention Study. Circulation. 2003 Jul 29;108(4):414-9.

53. https://food-guide.canada.ca/en/

54. Mozaffarian D, Katan MB, Ascherio A, Stampfer MJ, Willett WC. Trans fatty acids and cardiovascular disease. New England Journal of Medicine. 2006 Apr 13;354(15):1601-13.

55. Vogel RA, Corretti MC, and Plotnick GD. Effect of a single

high-fat meal on endothelial function in healthy subjects. Am J Cardiol 1997 (79):350-354.

56. Josse A, Kendall C, Augustin L, Ellis P, Jenkins D. Almonds decrease post-prandial glycemia—a dose response study. Metabolism 2007;56:400-4.

57. Lichtenstein A, Appel L, Brands M, et al. Diet and lifestyle recommendations revision 2006: a scientific statement from the American Heart Association Nutrition Committee. Circulation 2006;114:82-96.

58. Arora S, McFarlane S. The case for low carbohydrate diets in diabetes management. Nutr Metab 2005;2:16-24.

Chapter 4
Enlisting Lunch
Reducing the Risk of Diabetes

To Heal with Surgical Steel

"Your doctor sent me a copy of your most recent bloodwork," I mentioned, as I flipped open the chart and sat down in front of Marion and her husband. "Your fasting blood sugar level was 6.4—higher than I'd like to see it," I said, showing her the lab report, and circling the concerning number. "It confirms that you have borderline or pre-diabetes."

"What do you mean by *borderline* diabetes?" Marion asked with a puzzled tone. "I thought you either had diabetes or you didn't," she added, matter-of-factly.

"It means you're on your way," I replied. "Your body is giving you a heads up that it's having some difficulty controlling your blood sugar levels. This commonly occurs in people with high blood pressure and an increased waist circumference, and is all part of the metabolic syndrome."

"Oh, wonderful," she said sarcastically. "Borderline diabetes isn't enough; I have to get some syndrome thrown on top. Why's all this happening *now*? I don't eat much.

I hardly have anything for lunch, just a small salad, and sometimes nothing at all," Marion said, bewildered.

"You're not alone. Borderline diabetes and full-blown diabetes, for that matter, are very common in our society. Type 2 diabetes usually takes years to develop and occurs more commonly as we age," I answered.

"Yeah, I was diagnosed with diabetes about ten years ago," her husband offered up. "It really scared me. So, I went on a crash diet and lost a bunch of weight… and I was able to bring my sugar levels back to normal," he said triumphantly. "Of course, that was then. Over the past few years, I gained it all back, and now I'm on my diabetic medications again. I guess it's just a matter of time," he added with a sigh.

"Actually, it's not just a matter of *time*," I countered. "It's a matter of *tolerance*. Adult-onset diabetes develops after our bodies become less sensitive to the action of insulin—a phenomenon called impaired glucose tolerance. High sugar loads in our diet place high demands on insulin production and eventually can make our bodies less sensitive to the important action of insulin. Excess abdominal fat tends to accelerate the process and, if left unchecked, can lead to diabetes. But the good news is that, at this stage, it can be prevented and even reversed, as you demonstrated some years ago," I said encouragingly to Marion's husband.

"Is bariatric surgery helpful to prevent diabetes?" Marion asked hopefully. "I've heard that gastric banding surgery is the best way to take the pounds off and was wondering if it might be a good idea for me."

"Gastric banding and gastric bypass surgeries can foster significant weight loss and have been shown to reduce the risk of diabetes,"[55] I confirmed. "We could certainly consider some form of bariatric surgery for you, but you need to realize that surgery is not a stand-alone solution for weight management."

"I was afraid you were going to say that," Marion said with a smile.

"The problems associated with obesity and the underlying cardiovascular issues are far more complex than we can heal with surgical steel," I went on. "Sedentary behaviours coupled with high sugar and high-fat diets cause vascular injury that accelerates the atherosclerotic process, even after successful surgery. Weight management clinics, like the Weight Wise Program we have next door, are designed to help get at the root cause of weight gain. They involve an entire team of health professionals including nurses, dieticians, and exercise specialists, who develop strategies that not only assist with weight reduction but also set out a comprehensive lifestyle approach for healthy weight maintenance.[56]

Even for those select patients who go on to have bariatric surgery, such as gastric banding or gastric bypass, it's still critical that they incorporate healthy behaviours into their daily lives to keep their weight under control and their diabetes at bay," I explained.

"So, you're saying that gastric banding surgery isn't a cure-all?" Marion asked with a tone of disappointment.

"Not so much," I said honestly. "Besides, it doesn't make sense to rely solely upon surgery to address a problem caused by our lifestyles, and it's just not good medicine. If we're truly concerned about protecting our blood vessels from disease and preventing diabetes, we'll need to do more than surgically modify our digestive tracts. When it comes to vascular health, there is no free lunch. Every snack and every meal has the potential to harm or to heal. We need to choose wisely when and what we eat... lunch included," I said.

Never Say Diabetes

What do Neil Young, Mary Tyler Moore, Drew Carey, and Smokin' Joe Frazier all have in common? Yes, they're all celebrity icons, and except for Neil Young, they can all sing. But, there's something more: they each have diabetes. With over 240 million people worldwide who suffer from diabetes, it's an all too common problem.[57] Diabetes affects nearly one in four North Americans over the age of sixty years, and the prevalence is growing by epidemic proportions, increasing by over 60 percent since 1990. Epidemiologic studies project that the number will more than double by the year 2025 (fig. 4.1).[58] Considering that 80 percent of people with diabetes die of heart disease, the increasing prevalence of diabetes is a cardiovascular disaster in the making.

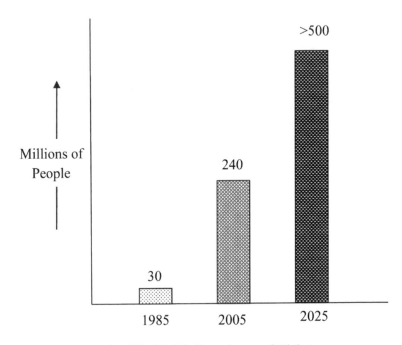

Fig. 4.1 Increasing Worldwide Prevalence of Diabetes

Diabetes refers to a group of diseases that cause high blood sugar levels. Most people with diabetes, about 90 percent of them, have what's called type 2 diabetes, a condition of our own making. This occurs when the body no longer responds to the important actions of insulin and is termed insulin resistant. As a result, blood sugar levels get all messed up, with no place to go but higher. It commonly occurs in people with increased abdominal fat and high blood pressure, like my patient Marion. By contrast, about 10 percent of people with diabetes have what's called type 1 diabetes. In this form of diabetes, there is an insufficient amount of insulin available to do the work. Type 1 diabetes is caused by the destruction of the insulin-producing organ, the pancreas, by the body's own immune system, leading to a state of insulin deficiency.

Nowadays, people with both type 1 and type 2 diabetes can continue to lead reasonably normal lives, but this wasn't the case even a century ago. Before the twenties got roaring, diabetes was a dreadful diagnosis to deliver. Telling a patient that their unexplained weight loss, complaints of thirst, need to urinate frequently, and malaise were because of type 1 diabetes was like saying, "I'm afraid you've got terminal cancer. I'm very sorry." Without any viable treatment, the diagnosis of type 1 diabetes used to be a death sentence. Within weeks of diagnosis, patients became emaciated, followed inevitably by diabetic coma and death. Strict attention to a meticulously regulated, calorie-restricted diet could buy a bit of time, but even the most diligent dieter succumbed within a year or two after receiving the deadly diagnosis. In the summer of 1921, Frederick Banting and Charles Best changed all that with their discovery of insulin. Today, with over fifty million people depending upon insulin to live another day, it's no wonder that the discovery of insulin is regarded by many as the single greatest medical breakthrough of all time.

Live and Let Diabetes

Unfortunately, the story of diabetes doesn't end with Banting and Best saddling up and riding off into the sunset, or with diabetic patients abandoning worry and living happily ever after—at least not as of yet. To be sure, the discovery of insulin changed the face of diabetes. With insulin therapy, blood sugar could enter into cells and be used as fuel, not left floating in circulation. As a result, children and teens were no longer wasting away from the consuming fire of diabetes, reduced to skin-covered skeletons, and succumbing to inescapable diabetic coma. This is truly a wonderful achievement. However, as life-saving as Banting and Best's discovery has proven to be, insulin is not a cure for diabetes. The injections do wonders to stabilize blood sugar levels and can permit those living with the disease to continue to do so, but insulin doesn't grant freedom from diabetes. Some critics go as far as to say that the discovery of insulin may have even hampered the finding of a cure for diabetes, but this is a bit harsh. Like Aesop's fox sneering at the sour grapes dangling on a branch out of reach, the comment was likely made by some sore loser, who was scooped by Banting.

All jealousy aside, one unfortunate result has come from the discovery of insulin. It has allowed for the relentless, inexorable, manifestation of the chronic complications associated with diabetes. In fact, before patients were saved with the advent of insulin therapy, no one would have dreamt just how much calamity the disease could cause. Rising blood sugar levels isn't the half of it. From head to toe, no limb or organ escapes its wrath. Diabetes is to modern medicine what syphilis must have been to medics before penicillin hit the market. Sir William Osler, renowned clinician and Chief of Staff at the Johns Hopkins Hospital in the 1890s, said to his medical students, "To know syphilis is to know medicine." Today, syphilis is curable with a single injection of an antibiotic, but diabetes carries on relentlessly, despite regular, carefully-adjusted, daily injections of insulin. Perhaps some statistics are to illustrate the extent and devastation of diabetic complications. Get comfortable and hold on tight, 'cause the list is long and the ride is wild.

Diabetes injures the blood vessels supplying the inner surface of the eye, or retina, and is the number one cause of blindness in North American adults, responsible for over 10,000 new cases of blindness every year in the United States alone;[59] diabetes causes kidney disease in 40 percent of diabetics, and is the leading cause of kidney failure and need for dialysis treatment in North America;[60] people with diabetes are twice as likely to develop high blood pressure, compared with people without diabetes,[61] and they are twenty-five times more likely to require amputation of a foot or leg due to circulatory problems related to diabetes;[62] nearly one-half of diabetic men will experience erectile dysfunction, or impotence, at some point in their lives;[63] and despite the many advances that have improved diabetic treatments, life expectancy for people with diabetes is reduced by ten to fifteen years below the average. Although the problems listed below (see fig. 4.2) are more commonly seen in patients with poorly-controlled diabetes, they can occur despite optimal, modern management. This sobering fact underscores the critical need to do more than prescribe medicines for diabetes; we need to do all we can to prevent this disease from getting any foothold.

Blindness
Slowed digestion (gastroparesis)
Kidney failure
Increased susceptibility to infection
Delayed healing capacity
Impotence (erectile dysfunction)
Urinary retention and incontinence
Peripheral nerve damage (neuropathy)
Joint deformity
Foot ulceration
Lower limb amputation

Fig. 4.2 Complications of Diabetes

The reason that diabetes causes such widespread havoc in the body is that it's a vascular disease. The earliest pathological effects of diabetes show up in the vascular cells that directly encounter elevated blood sugar levels. Diabetes injures our blood vessels by damaging the inner lining, inciting vascular inflammation underneath the lining, and fostering cholesterol accumulation deep within blood vessel walls (fig. 4.3). This injury involves all blood vessels, large and small, day and night, for richer and for poorer, 'till death do you part. And since blood vessels go everywhere in our body, so can the talons of diabetes.

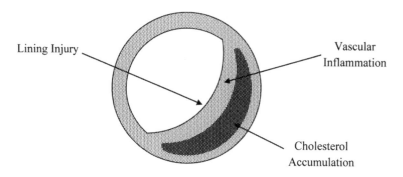

Fig. 4.3 Diabetes Injures Blood Vessels

Not surprisingly then, the major cause of death in patients with type 2 diabetes (the adult-onset, acquired variety) is cardiovascular in nature, including sudden cardiac death, heart attack, heart failure, and stroke.[64] Studies have shown that the heart attack risk for someone with diabetes is the same as it is for someone who has established heart artery disease.[65] One-half of heart attack patients have elevated blood sugar levels, and they're the half that don't do as well, with an almost fourfold increased prospect of dying in the hospital compared with patients without diabetes or elevated blood sugar levels.[66] As well, compared with the general population, patients with diabetes have two to three times the risk of stroke, which accounts for 20 percent of all deaths in diabetic patients.[67] Considering that stroke is the second most frequent cause of death worldwide and the most frequent cause of permanent disability, that's a whole lot of trouble. Diabetes also erases the gender protection from heart attack and stroke behind which pre-menopausal women take shelter.[68] In other words, from a vascular perspective, when a woman develops diabetes, her blood vessels become as prone to atherosclerotic disease as a man's. Gender equality is a wonderful thing, except when it comes to cardiovascular disease.

Arriving at the Diagnosis

There is no time to delay. Since some of the vascular injuries caused by diabetes can be reduced, and even reversed, it's important to make the diagnosis of diabetes as soon as possible. So, to minimize the time between the onset of pre-diabetes (or borderline diabetes), and the occurrence of blood vessel injury, we need to be looking for diabetes before obvious complications arise. The Canadian Diabetes Association recommends routine screening for type 2 diabetes every three years for those over forty years of age with any of the risk factors listed below (Table 4.1), or with diabetes-associated conditions.[69] Do yourself a favour and get tested. You may not have any symptoms or signs as of yet, but if your blood sugar level is high, you'll at least be aware that you've got to make some immediate changes to ward off the full-fledged disease.

G	Gestational Diabetes (history of diabetes occurring during pregnancy)
L	Living with heart disease or stroke (known vascular disease)
U	Upwards of 40 years old
C	Cholesterol elevation
O	Overweight
S	Sibling or parent (family history of diabetes)
E	Elevated blood pressure

Table 4.1 GLUCOSE Risk Factors for Type 2 Diabetes

The two tests that are commonly utilized to confirm the diagnosis of diabetes are the fasting blood glucose test (FBG), as Marion had done, and the more precise oral glucose tolerance test (OGTT). Both tests require that you refrain from eating or drinking for at least eight hours. The fasting blood glucose test is then just a single needle poke and you're done. A blood sugar level between 6.1 and 6.9 mmol/L suggests borderline, or pre-diabetes, and a result of 7.0 or above meets the diagnostic criteria for diabetes. The oral glucose tolerance test is used to confirm the FBG test result and to identify those individuals who may still have pre-diabetes, despite having near-normal fasting blood sugar levels (that is, those with fasting blood glucose levels in the grey zone of 5.6-6.0 mmol/L). The OGTT is a little more cumbersome a test, requiring two blood tests two hours apart. After the first fasting blood sugar sample is taken, you have to drink a sickly sweet sugar solution, containing 75 grams of sugar. Then, after two hours of reading *People Magazine* or *Reader's Digest,* a second sample is drawn. The results can separate out those who have normal sugar metabolism from those with either pre-diabetes or full-blown diabetes (see table 4.2). You may feel fine, but you could still have undiagnosed diabetes or pre-diabetes. The concern about pre-diabetes isn't just the heightened risk of developing overt diabetes, although 25 percent of people with pre-diabetes will do so. Pre-diabetes significantly increases the risk of cardiovascular disease.[70] So, why not ask your doctor about getting tested? When it comes to diabetes and its many serious complications, ignorance isn't bliss, and it might just prove to be the kiss of death.

Status	8-Hour Fasting Blood Glucose (mmol/L)	2-Hour Oral Glucose Tolerance Test (mmol/L)
Normal	< 6.1	< 7.8
Pre-Diabetes	6.1 - 6.9 (Impaired Fasting Glucose)	7.8 - 11.1 (Impaired Glucose Tolerance)
Diabetes Mellitus	> 7.0	> 11.1

Table 4.2 Diagnostic Criteria for Diabetes and Pre-Diabetes

Transplantation for the Nation?

Research teams are continuing to strive towards a cure for diabetes. Pancreas transplantation is a particularly exciting option for patients with type 1 diabetes (who have insufficient insulin production), allowing them to once again naturally make and secrete their own insulin, independent of daily self-injections. But such an approach is not without risk. Excessive bleeding, infection, and organ rejection are but a few of the potentially life-threatening complications associated with transplantation surgery.[71] And since people with diabetes are already more prone to infections because of compromised immune systems, the use of lifelong medications to prevent rejection of the transplanted pancreas (immunosuppressive therapy), adds significant complexity to their management. As a result, pancreas transplantation isn't appropriate for all patients with type 1 diabetes but is reserved for a select few: those patients who have extreme difficulty in regulating their blood sugar levels (a condition called brittle diabetes), and those who have renal failure and are undergoing kidney transplantation. These latter patients will need to take lifelong immunosuppressive therapy for their transplanted kidneys, anyway, so combining the procedure with pancreas transplantation makes good sense.

Refinements in pancreas transplantation include using just pancreas fragments, rather than the entire organ; that is, transplanting the insulin-producing portion of the pancreas from a deceased donor into a patient with type 1 diabetes. The Edmonton Protocol, a type of islet cell transplant developed in 1999 by Dr. James Shapiro at the University of Alberta (Canada), uses a unique islet-cell preparation technique and immunosuppressant-drug regimen and has dramatically improved success rates of this approach.[72]

Unfortunately, patients who receive islet-cell transplants often still require regular, supplemental insulin injections for optimal blood sugar control. So, although the procedure can protect diabetic patients from extreme blood sugar fluctuations, insulin adjustments remain a ball and chain.

Significant medical advances have also taken place for patients with type 2 diabetes (who are resistant to the action of insulin). During the last few years, new blood sugar lowering drugs have been added to the diabetic drug armamentarium; including such unpronounceable medicines as exenatide, sitagliptin, and vildagliptin. Acting on novel metabolic pathways, these and other currently available medicines not only improve blood sugar levels, but they also increase the body's sensitivity to insulin and reduce the likelihood of type 2 diabetic patients requiring insulin injections.[73] Such therapies, coupled with close attention to blood pressure and cholesterol control, can improve the quality of life for people with type 2 diabetes. However, medicines don't address the underlying cause of the metabolic difficulties that predispose to diabetes, namely increased abdominal fat. Like treating sleep deprivation with a pot of morning coffee, or fixing your kitchen sink with duct tape, these medications may provide some benefits in the short term, but they do nothing to address the excess bodyweight causing insulin resistance. If we want to better manage existing diabetes, or better yet, prevent diabetes from developing in the first place, we can't ignore the central role that bodyweight plays in blood sugar control.

It's Do or Diabetes

Type 2 diabetes is largely preventable. Studies have repeatedly shown that lifestyle interventions aimed at reducing abdominal fat can not only stall the onset of type 2 diabetes but prevent the whole metabolic mess from getting started in the first place.[74] This has been demonstrated across all ethnic backgrounds and in both men and women. Even high-risk individuals, like Marion, who already have borderline diabetes can successfully navigate back to the safety of healthy blood sugar levels if they act swiftly. The magnitude of lifestyle changes required to significantly reduce the risk of developing diabetes doesn't have to be drastic. As little as a 5 percent reduction in weight is enough to get the ball rolling in the right direction. Within short months of losing this amount of weight, the risk of developing overt diabetes can be slashed by a whopping 50 percent. Sounds like an irresistible Boxing Day Sale, doesn't it? But here's the difference. We're not talking about buying more unnecessary stuff that will collect dust in your basement. Preventing diabetes is about preventing vascular disease, including heart disease and stroke.

To best achieve this 5 percent drop in weight and reduce the risk of developing diabetes, there are two recommended interventions. First, a reduction in the daily amount of ingested fatty foods, particularly animal fats (saturated) and processed fats (trans-fats); and second, an increase in the amount of daily physical activity. One conclusive study from Finland followed 522 middle-aged, overweight subjects (172 men and 350 women, with a mean age of 55 years) who had impaired glucose tolerance, over a six-year period. Half the group received individualized health counselling and the other half did not. The counselling included dietary recommendations aimed at reducing fat ingestion, as well as information on exercise strategies. They asked participants to take part in at least four hours of physical activity per week, which could include a variety of things, from biking or swimming, to walking or gardening. Within the first year of study, the intervention group lost an average of five kilograms of weight (11 lbs), while the control group lost less than one kilogram (2 lbs). But even though the difference in weight reduction between the two groups was only a modest amount, the risk of developing diabetes was strikingly different. The lifestyle intervention group, armed with only dietary and activity modifications, demonstrated a remarkable 58 percent reduction in the incidence of type 2 diabetes (fig. 4.4),[75] underscoring the utmost importance of this simple strategy.

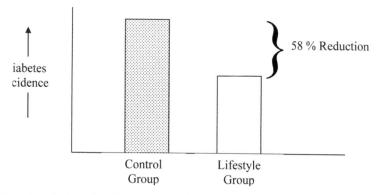

Fig. 4.4 Lifestyle Changes Reduce the Risk of Developing Diabetes

Lunch Liberation

There is no need to be oppressed by the gloomy prospect of developing diabetes. We can be freed from needless worrying by giving some serious thought to lifestyle changes and earnestly incorporating them into our daily lives. The lunch hour is an ideal time to implement these ideas. It might take a little creative thought, but reducing fat ingestion and getting active during the lunch break shouldn't represent an impossible mission. Besides, the health benefits are well worth the effort. Not only can we reduce our risk of developing the dreaded diabetes, but these changes are also central to weight loss, they will improve our vascular health, and they can even help counter that annoying afternoon energy slump, all in one fell swoop. Start by considering your lunch options. Do you really need to go to Sammy's Decadent Diner or the All-You-Can-Eat Golden Dragon

Buffet at noon? Wouldn't it be more efficient, and less expensive, to bring something healthier from home to eat for lunch? If we're serious about our health in general and our heart health in particular, we need to go lean on lunch. So, forget French fries, chicken nuggets, poutine, burgers, creamy soups and creamy salads. Regardless of the status of our wallets, our tummies certainly can't afford any of these options. And why should they? There are plenty of lean lunch ideas that can meet our nutritional needs and not add to our abdominal adipose (fig. 4.5). With a little planning, ideally the night before, we can avoid unnecessary fat consumption during lunch and better protect ourselves from the wrath of diabetes.

Hummus and pita bread with some crudités (bite-sized raw veggies)
Chickpea and tuna salad
Grilled chicken breast sliced onto greens
Salmon lettuce whole-wheat wrap
Minestrone with half a slice of multigrain bread
Turkey chili on brown rice
Vegetarian lasagna filled with cottage cheese

Fig. 4.5 Leaner Lunch Suggestions

Choosing lean options for your lunch box isn't enough to reduce the risk of diabetes; we need to get active, as well, and the lunch hour is an ideal time to do so. All work and no play not only make Johnny a dull boy, but it also fosters insulin resistance and increases the risk of diabetes. In addition to dietary modification, studies have consistently demonstrated that the interventions which include exercise regimens as part of the lifestyle recommendations are the most effective in reducing the likelihood of those with borderline diabetes from developing overt diabetes, even better than medications can.[76] No one can afford to let this opportunity pass them by. Although the beneficial mechanisms of exercise on blood sugar metabolism are complex, they can be considered in this simplified fashion: everything that diabetes does to injure our blood vessels—damaging the blood vessel lining, fanning vascular-wall inflammation and augmenting cholesterol accumulation within our arteries—is countered by regular exercise. This means that by simply stretching our legs and taking in some fresh air over the lunch hour, we can help to mitigate the mischief that high blood sugar levels can inflict on our blood vessels.[77] No matter what our age or our current fitness level, as little as twenty-five minutes of walking a day has been shown to improve insulin sensitivity and postpone the development of diabetes.[78] This amount of walking can also help to whittle away at Health Canada's recommended 60 to 90 minutes of daily physical activity. If you're searching for a sure-fire way to improve blood sugar control, assist with weight maintenance, and reduce the risk of heart disease and stroke, look no further than your Reeboks, and choose a walking lunch over a working lunch.

Timing Lunchtime

Each day our heart beats over 100,000 times, pushing over half a million litres of blood through over 100,000 kilometres of snaking vessels, and we take about 26,000 breaths, moving some 14,000 litres of air in and out of our lungs. It's a bit of work, and it all requires energy. As a result of this steady demand, our bodies are designed to conserve energy, so that we can, at the very least, maintain these vital functions. From a developmental perspective of our species, this is very important. Considering the recurring cycles of famine that have plagued humankind, stretching out over history like my boys' handprints across our front picture window, it stands to reason that such a safeguard is firmly established. If our bodies were as wastefully extravagant with energy as our homes and vehicles are, there's no way we could've survived the lean years of the past. Even Joseph, with his *Amazing Technicolor Dreamcoat*, and his sage advice for Pharaoh to layaway grain for drought insurance, couldn't have saved us from starving through the centuries.

The idea that we have a genetic default setting that is geared toward net energy conservation is called the *Thrifty Gene Hypothesis*. It's thought to be a built-in survival mechanism and it goes something like this: during the all-you-can-eat times of plenty, we store energy, in the form of abdominal fat, to prepare for the leaner times of peas and parsnips that may potentially lie ahead. Then, during those actual leaner times, our bodies conserve energy by slowing our metabolism.

If we eat erratically and allow serendipity to guide our food choices, we are more likely to make the wrong choices, choosing energy-dense items that are too heavy on fat, salt and sugar, and too light on nutrition. We need to beware; our unsatisfied appetites prowl around like roaring lions, seeking a moment of weakness to strike. When we don't eat at regular times in the day, we make ourselves vulnerable to such an attack. Try as we might, it's difficult to escape the food advertisers' propaganda telling us to eat all the time, if for no other reason than to indulge ourselves. The food industry's giant advertising machine is primed and ready to catch us in our moments of weakness, flaunting giant close-ups of French fries on billboards and buses, full-page glossy magazine photos of sundaes and sauces, and seductive television commercials of cascading, swirling, milk chocolate rivers. It's a jungle of temptation out there and inconsistent eating behaviour leads us into the middle of it, like a lamb to the slaughter. It's hard to say "No" to junk food when it's staring us in the face and doubly hard when our stomachs are grumbling. A healthy lunch choice can provide just the protection we need, when we need it most.

Skirting the Slippery Slump

One annoying consequence of making a poor lunch choice comes two or three hours later. No, I'm not referring to the nausea from eating all six spring rolls, or the heartburn from the chilli-pepper pizza; but rather the annoying afternoon energy slump. As predictable as sunshine on the Sahara, the wrath of drowsiness is sure to visit you as 2 or 3 p.m. rolls around. Despite our caffeine-centred culture, a mid-afternoon energy slump is a recurring event for most, and a daily struggle for many. The experience can be most unpleasant. Consider yesterday afternoon, for example. After you got back from eating lunch at the Burger Baron and cleaned as much of the grease as you could from the stain on your lapel, you sat down at your desk to give some attention to your overdue project. Then, out of a clear blue sky, a yawn spread across your face and *wham-bam*, before you could say Rip Van Winkle, you slammed smack-dab into an impassable wall of fatigue and felt as though your life's blood had been drained from your limbs. You staggered in a haze to the staff room for a cup of caffeine rescue, when your colleague reminded you of the staff meeting. So, there you sat, eyes glazed over, listening to your boss's monotone state of the union address, pinching yourself till red welts formed on your thighs to keep from nodding off.

Do you ever wonder why this mid-afternoon energy slump arrives so predictably in the mid-afternoon? Could it be the re-circulated air wafting through the office, the energy-inefficient fluorescent light bulbs shining overhead, or perhaps the tug of our orbiting moon pulling on your brain? Some might think so, but the cause is more likely due to some of the culprits below, aligning like the planets to spell afternoon doom (table 4.2).

Too Little	Too Much
Sleep last night	Calorie consumption at lunch
Activity today	Salt and fat-laden processed food
Fluids on board	Refined carbohydrates
Lunch food energy	Caffeine

Table 4.3 Causes of the Afternoon Slump

I've subdivided common causes of the afternoon slump into a "too little" group and a "too much" group. If your afternoon fatigue is because of one or more of the items listed in the "too little" category, then good news; the solution is straightforward enough. Simply bang back a tall glass of water, eat an apple, perhaps along with a small handful of roasted almonds, take a fiver with eyes shut on the staff room couch, and then volunteer to take the office mail downstairs (using the stairs, both down and back up), and *voilà*! You'll be wide awake and ready to finish your workday with all the vim and vigour you crave. If, however, you slept well last night, ate all your lunch (even the raw broccoli and cauliflower florets), you didn't wait for thirst to set in but kept up on your fluids (eight glasses of water, that is, and lattes don't count), you've just come back from your noon walk around the block, and despite all this, you're still falling over yourself with fatigue—well, then your slump issues are more likely due to something in the "too much" bin. If this is the case, the solution to your afternoon somnolence will require some cutting back and some planning ahead. Don't forget, even a healthy meal choice can make you nod off in the afternoon if the portion size was too sizeable. It's reminiscent of the "Oxygen" song by Sweet: Lunch "is like oxygen / you get too much, you get too high / not enough and you're gonna die." If you've gotten too much at lunch, there may be no quick fix for reducing your fatigue at this very moment. But, as Annie says, "tomorrow is just a day away." If you cut back on calories, salt, simple carbohydrates, and caffeine, then tomorrow can potentially be the first day of the rest of your slump-free life, and you can bet your bottom dollar that you'll have more energy.

Addressing this afternoon fatigue is important since it's not just our daytime wakefulness that's on the line here; it's our cardiovascular health. Taking some intentional measures to counter the afternoon energy slump by adding to the "too little" list or by subtracting from the "too much" list will have the added benefit of also improving the health of your heart and blood vessels. Conversely, by stubbornly trying to battle through the mid-afternoon malaise, eating another plate of chocolate cookies or drinking another triple-shot cappuccino, you'll be merely adding insult to vasculature injury and doing precious little to improve your wakefulness.[80] If you want to reduce the risk of heart disease and stroke, as well as control weight and prevent diabetes, you need to plan ahead and choose wisely from the lunch menu. By not dealing with the afternoon slump, the problem won't be just one of afternoon lethargy; it will be weight gain, metabolic strain, glucose intolerance, diabetes, and vascular catastrophe.

Thinking Outside the Lunch Box

"Are you saying that I should eat more for lunch?" Marion asked with a puzzled look. "I'm trying to *lose* weight, not *gain* it," she said, emphasizing her words as if I were hearing impaired, or a few cards short of a deck.

"Well, you need something more than just a few greens," I argued. "Add some lean protein like chicken breast or tuna next time. We must provide our bodies with sufficient, regularly-timed, nutritional calories throughout the day. It makes for steadier blood sugar levels, happier blood vessels, and more successful weight control efforts," I said.

"There's not much in the way of food options where I work and I don't have time for a formal, sit-down affair. I use my lunch hour to catch up on work; so, I need something fast and simple to eat for lunch," Marion explained.

"Join the club. Gone are the days of the two martini lunches, and just as well; after all, they just make a person see double and feel single," I responded with a grin. "I try to solve my 'what to have for lunch' dilemma the night before. I usually put some leftovers from dinner into a Tupperware container. In the morning, I pack it into my insulated lunch bag with some assorted fresh fruits and vegetables, and I'm good to go," I said.

"We don't usually have much for leftovers in our house.

By the time seconds are done, so is the meal," Marion smiled.

"Slowing down a tad to let your stomach catch up to your eyes can help stretch out the first helping... and drinking plenty of water, too. Because, make no mistake, those who eat seconds at a meal are the first to lose out on weight control," I cautioned. "My wife intentionally makes a double quantity of dinner. And even before we sit down to eat, she's already divvied up several individual-sized meal portions into Ziploc containers for our next day lunches," I explained.

"Sounds too organized for me," Marion surrendered.

"Weight management, time management, and even money management all go together. Bringing a lunch to work not only spares me from making unhealthy meal choices during the day, but it also saves me time and money, as well. When noon hour comes, a well-balanced, nutritious meal is just a nuke in the microwave away. It's so time-efficient that I can use part of my lunch hour to go for a walk. Stretching my legs and breathing some fresh air helps me beat the afternoon energy slump," I said. "If used well, the lunch hour is a perfect opportunity to burn some calories, build heart health, and help counter blood sugar mayhem."

Chapter Summary
Enlisting Lunch

- Diabetes is common and on the rise, affecting nearly one in four North Americans over the age of sixty

- Diabetes causes a long list of medical problems, including kidney disease, and increases the risk of sudden cardiac death, heart attack, heart failure, and stroke

- The acronym GLUCOSE includes the risk factors for developing type-2 diabetes and includes: Gestational diabetes; Living with vascular disease; Upwards of 40 years old; Cholesterol elevation; Overweight; Sibling or parent with diabetes; and Elevated blood pressure

- Most people with diabetes have type-2 adult-onset variety related to insulin resistance

- Lifestyle adaptations including exercise and a prudent diet have been shown to effectively counter insulin resistance

- Prevent the afternoon energy slump by drinking water, eating a lean lunch, doing some activity, and avoiding refined carbs or fat-laden lunches and too much caffeine

- Lean lunch options can help with weight control and reduce insulin resistance

- Homemade lunches provide healthier options than

eating out

- The lunch hour is a potential time for physical activity, which can burn calories, assist fitness, and help counter diabetes

Chapter Notes

59. Dixon JB, O'Brien PE, Playfair J, Chapman L, Schachter LM, Skinner S, Proietto J, Bailey M, Anderson M. Adjustable gastric banding and conventional therapy for type 2 diabetes: a randomized control trial. JAMA 2008;299 (3):316-23.

60. Obesity management. Eckel RH, Clinical practice. Nonsurgical management of obesity in adults. N Engl J Med. 2008;358:1941-1950.

61. Adeghate E, Schattner P, Dunn E. An update on the etiology and epidemiology of diabetes mellitus. Ann N Y Acad Sci. 2006 Nov;1084:1-29.

62. Lloyd-Jones D, Adams R, Carnethon M, et al. Heart disease and stroke statistics: 2009 Update. A report from the American Heart Association Statistics Committee and Stroke Statistics Subcommittee. Circulation 2009;119:e21-181.

63. Fong DS, Aiello LP, Ferris FL 3rd, Klein R: Diabetic retinopathy. Diabetes Care 2004; 27:2540 -2553.

64. Gross JL, de Azevedo MJ, Silveiro SP, Canani LH, Caramori ML, Zelmanovitz T: Diabetic nephropathy: diagnosis, prevention, and treatment. Diabetes Care 2005; 28: 164-176.

65. Fox CS, Coady S, Sorlie PD, et al. Increasing cardiovascular disease burden due to diabetes mellitus: the Framingham Heart Study. Circulation 2007;115:1544-1550.

66. Abbott CA et al. The North-West Diabetes Foot Care Study: incidence of, and risk factors for, new diabetic foot ulceration

in a community-based patient cohort. Diabet Med 2002;19 : 377-384.

67. M. J. Fowler. Microvascular and Macrovascular Complications of Diabetes. Clin. Diabetes, April 1, 2008; 26(2): 77 - 82.

68. Duckworth W, Abraira C, Moritz T, Reda D, Emanuele N, Reaven PD, Zieve FJ, Marks J, Davis SN, Hayward R, Warren SR, Goldman S, McCarren M, Vitek ME, Henderson WG, Huang GD. Glucose Control and Vascular Complications in Veterans with Type 2 DiabetesN Engl J Med 2009; 360:129-139.

69. Haffner S, Legto S, Onnemaa T, Pyorala K, Laakso M. Mortality from coronary heart disease in subjects with type 2 diabetes and in non-diabetic subjects with and without prior myocardial infarction. N Engl J Med 1998;339:229-234.

70. Donahoe SM, Stewart GC, McCabe CH, et al. Admission glucose and mortality in elderly patients hospitalized with acute myocardial infarction: implications for patients with and without recognized diabetes. Circulation 2005;111:3078-86.

71. D. Sander, K. Sander, and H. Poppert. Review: Stroke in type 2 diabetes. The British Journal of Diabetes & Vascular Disease, September 1, 2008; 8(5): 222—229.

72. Engberding N, Wenger NK. Cardiovascular disease prevention tailored for women. Expert Rev Cardiovasc Ther. 2008 Sep;6(8):1123-34.

73. Canadian Diabetes Association 2008 Clinical Practice Guidelines for the Prevention and Management of Diabetes in Canada. Canadian Journal of Diabetes 2008;32(Suppl 1) S1-S201.

74. Ritz E. Total cardiovascular risk management. Am J Cardiol. 2007 Aug 6;100(3A):53J-60J.

75. Reddy, K.S. et al. Long-term survival following simultaneous

kidney-pancreas transplantation versus kidney transplantation alone in patients with type 1 diabetes mellitus and renal failure. American Journal of Kidney Disease 2003;41: 464–70.

76. Shapiro J, Ricordi C, Hering BJ,et al. International Trial of the Edmonton Protocol for Islet Transplantation. N Engl J Med 2006;355(13):1318-1330.

77. Srinivasan BT, Jarvis J, Khunti K, Davies MJ. Recent advances in the management of type 2 diabetes mellitus: a review. Postgraduate Medical Journal 2008;84:524-531.

78. Horton ES. Effects of lifestyle changes to reduce risks and associated cardiovascular risks: results from large scale efficacy trials. Obesity. Dec 2009;Suppl 3:S43-8.

79. Tuomilehto J, Lindstrom J, Eriksson JG, Valle TT, et al. Finnish Diabetes Prevention Study Group. Prevention of type 2 diabetes mellitus by changes in lifestyle among subjects with impaired glucose tolerance. N Engl J Med 2001;344(18):1343-50.

80. Zimmet P, Shaw J, Alberti KGMM. Preventing Type 2 diabetes and the dysmetabolic syndrome in the real world: a realistic view. Diabetic Medicine 2003;20(9):693-702.

81. Houmard JA, Tanner CJ, Slentz CA, Duscha BD, McCartney JS, Kraus WE. Effect of the volume and intensity of exercise training on insulin sensitivity. J Appl Physiol. 2004 Jan;96(1):101-6.

82. Kirwan JP, Kohrt WM, Wojta DM, Bourey RE, Holloszy JO. Endurance exercise training reduces glucose-stimulated insulin levels in 60- to 70-year-old men and women. J Gerontol. 1993 May;48(3):M84-90.

83. Anderson C, Horne JA. A high sugar content, low caffeine drink does not alleviate sleepiness but may worsen it. Hum Psychopharmacol. 2006 Jul;21(5):299-303.

Chapter 5
Fitness Trumps Fatness
Benefits of Full-body Fitness

Marion's Worthy Risk

"I've really been dreading this," Marion said, as I joined her in the exercise stress lab. "And it didn't help matters when your nurse told me that there's a risk!" she complained.

"Yes, exercise stress testing does pose a small risk of heart attack, stroke, or death,[84] but no different than if you were walking along the trails in the river valley," I said, pointing out the window. "And it's a risk worth taking," I added. "With your risk factors and your family history of heart trouble, I think it's important for us to check your response to exercise and see if there's anything to suggest inadequate blood supply to your heart muscle. The risk of not knowing this is far greater than the risk of walking on the treadmill," I said.

"It's just that you hear about people dropping dead when they're exercising—even athletes," Marion said anxiously.

"Fortunately, that's not very often. And it's not usually the exercise that's to blame; more often than not, exercise is merely the trigger. Sudden deaths that occur with exertion are typically because of some underlying heart abnormality. For the athlete, that abnormality is usually a structural anomaly or some electrical wiring problem. For non-athletic types, it's usually heart artery disease—my very concern for you," I said. "So, come on. Let's check things out," I said, inviting her forward to start the test.

"Well, I guess if I'm going to have a heart attack, it may as well be here," Marion said in surrender, as she stepped onto the treadmill platform.

"I'll start you off nice and slow—just as if you were walking down the hallway at home," I said, as I started the belt and adjusted the speed. "And now for some interest, here's a bit of a hill," I added, and increased the treadmill incline in accordance with Stage 1 of our exercise protocol.

"Why is it that exercising increases the risk of heart attacks? I thought it was supposed to be healthy for you," Marion asked, as she relaxed into her stride.

"All of us have some degree of fat build-up within the walls of our blood vessels," I said in response. "When we exercise, the force on our blood vessel walls increases and can potentially cause an unstable plaque with a large cholesterol core to crack open and rupture," I explained. "Usually, it's the sudden bursts of activity that get people into trouble; the kind with no warm-up or cool-down. Snow shoveling is the classic scenario. But for those of us who make exercise a regular part of each day, the risk of heart trouble during exertion—while not zero—is very low. Habitual exercise helps remove cholesterol from our blood vessel walls and, as a result, can significantly decrease the risk of sudden death during the twenty-four hours or so that follow a workout (fig.5.1).[85] Benchwarmers don't enjoy that kind of benefit," I said encouragingly.

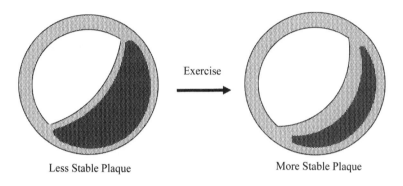

Less Stable Plaque   More Stable Plaque

Fig. 5.1 Exercise Stabilizes Vascular Plaques

"Am I done yet?" Marion whined.

"Not quite. For best results from this test, we need to increase your heart rate into the target zone," I explained, pointing to her heart rate readout on the monitor. "So, the treadmill's going to get a little faster and steeper now," I warned, as she completed her first three minutes and entered the second stage of the exercise protocol.

"Oh boy!" she said, surprised by the increased workload. "I'm not sure how long I can do this for."

"Well, I was going to go downstairs for a coffee. I'll check back with you later this afternoon," I teased.

"Oh, no you don't," she said. "If I'm going down, I want you catching me," she smiled, as she stepped up to the challenge.

The Risk of Sitting Around

Many think that watching is safer than doing, but it's not so; spectators are also at risk. I don't mean the risk of a wild slap shot careening over the protective glass into the blue section at a hockey game, or a foul ball flying into the middle of the fan-filled baseball stadium. Keep on the lookout for projectile possibilities, certainly, but I'm referring to something far more common and far more life-threatening. Out of a clear blue sky, people who lead sedentary lives can be struck by heart attacks and stroke. In fact, sitting is now recognized as an independent risk factor for all-cause mortality and developing cardiovascular disease. This was illustrated at the 2006 World Cup FIFA (French for International Federation of Association Football) Championship in Germany. It was when hundreds of thousands of sedentary spectators (in dire need of some exercise) watched thirty-two competing teams (in dire need of some rest). Despite the intense competition, no soccer player suffered a heart attack or stroke during the tournaments. However, the same could not be said for the spectators. As it turned out, the fans watching the soccer tournament had a more than doubled risk of heart attack above population norms.[86] There is no safe seat when it comes to heart disease, particularly in the bleachers. Epidemiological studies have shown that sedentary elderly men have twice the mortality rate as an age-matched cohort who walked two miles or more per day.[87] The same is true for women. In the Nurses' Health Study, which included over 70,000 women between the ages of forty and sixty-five, there was a strong, graded relationship between activity level and heart health; those who were most sedentary had the highest risk of heart disease and stroke, and those who were most active had the least risk.[88] It's been shown that sedentary behaviour carries a risk of heart attack similar to smoking a pack of cigarettes every day.[89] As a result, in 1996 The American Heart Association listed a sedentary lifestyle as an independent risk factor for developing premature cardiovascular disease. Since an estimated 60 percent of Canadians are physically inactive, a higher prevalence than for any other major cardiovascular risk factor, sedentary behaviour is an enormous challenge facing our nation's health.[90]

While physicians may be well-positioned to address this challenge of sedentary behaviour by cheerleading our patients into active living, we seldom do. Giving practical, individualized exercise advice with patients takes time. Given the six and a half minutes, on average, which family physicians spend with their patients, it's difficult to even scratch the surface of the topic. Suggesting to a patient that "You need to go out and exercise," is of no more value than saying, "Have a nice day." They've heard it all before. Another reason that physicians may be reluctant to discuss exercise with their patients is their comfort level with the topic. The lion's share of a doctor's training is devoted to the detection and management of disease, not the optimization and maintenance of health. So, when it comes to the issue of sudden cardiac death, our undivided attention naturally gets focused on high-risk patients. This includes those people who have had a prior heart attack and suffer from reduced heart pump function, as well as those with documented serious heart rhythm disorders.

Despite the impressive advances in cardiovascular medicine, such as the development of implantable defibrillators (a specialized pacemaker that delivers an electrical shock to the patient in the event of a life-threatening heart rhythm occurrence), high technology has had a negligible effect on the sudden cardiac death statistics. This is because the majority of sudden cardiac deaths involve the general population—ordinary folks like you and me.[91] One third of heart-related deaths happen suddenly—most within the first hour of symptoms, the majority of which occur in people without a prior history of heart disease.[92] Last year there were over 300,000 sudden cardiac deaths in North America and only a small fraction involved high-risk patients (fig. 5.2).[93]

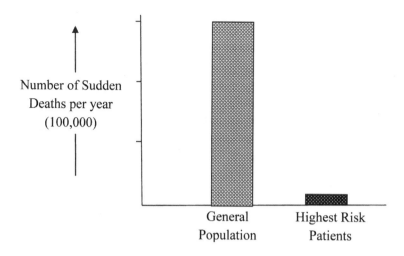

Fig. 5.2 Incidence of Sudden Cardiac Death

For those of us over the age of thirty-five, sudden cardiac death is most commonly related to atherosclerotic plaque buildup on the inside of our arteries. Since exercise is a proven effective means of reducing plaque buildup, if we want to reduce sudden death rates, encouraging daily exercise is a good place to start. When it comes to cardiovascular risk, it's not better to let sleeping dogs lie. Our dogs need exercise, and so do we.

Although it's sometimes difficult to avoid, sedentary behaviour is dangerous and needs to be countered. When I know that I've got a sedentary stretch coming, like a long flight or series of unavoidable meetings, I purposely plan some resistance exercise beforehand. It makes the rest feel more deserved, and the sitting time gives the muscles a chance to recover. The more sedentary our work is, the more intentional we need to be about incorporating exercise into our week. Take my clinical work, for example. I spend hours on end reading echocardiogram studies, electrocardiograms, and Holter monitor reports, and hours again making phone calls and wading through piles of paperwork, and all the while sitting. Recognizing the dangers of this, I plan exercise times into the white space of my week. I have to be pretty creative sometimes, like doing an early morning weight routine before ward rounds or using a portion of my lunch-hour to do a stair workout in the hospital stairwell. On nice days, I bike to work instead of driving. To avoid rush hour, I go for a late-afternoon jog through the neighborhood next to the hospital, or if its winter, I do some cross-country skiing in the River Valley on the way home, and then plan a later dinner. It sure beats the bumper-to-bumper traffic and allows me to redeem the day from a fitness standpoint.

Made Marion Move it

"The treadmill is going to get a little faster in about ten seconds," I said to Marion as she was finishing the second stage of the exercise protocol. "What do you think? Do you want to try the next level?" I asked, with my finger hovering over the "recovery" button just in case she decided to be done.

"No, I don't think so," she gasped. "Any faster and I won't be able to keep up!" she said in submission, with a pained look on her face.

"Fair enough," I said and immediately reduced the treadmill speed to a comfortable walking pace, allowing her time to cool down. "That wasn't so bad, now was it?" I asked.

"Maybe not for you," Marion retorted. "But, I'm exhausted. Did you see anything wrong?"

"No, it looks fine. There's nothing worrisome on the electrocardiogram to suggest a blood flow problem," I said reassuringly. "Did you have any chest discomfort or pressure during the test?" I asked as I assisted her back to the chair.

"No, I'm just short of breath," she said, still visibly winded.

"All you need now," I said, using my cheerleading tone, "is a decent pair of walking shoes and thirty minutes a day to use them."

"Well, I'm not sure my knees can handle too much walking," she said hesitantly. "Besides," it's too cold and icy outside."

"Although I try to avoid the really cold days, too, the weather usually doesn't slow me down much," I countered. "My dog has her eyes fixed on me the moment I get home from work and she doesn't give me a moment's peace until I've taken her for our daily jaunt. But, there are more ways to improve your fitness level than just walking. The sky's the limit when it comes to indoor exercise options—swimming, biking, rowing, striding on an elliptical trainer, or mastering a StairMaster—and all excellent choices for minimizing joint trauma. I've got a stationary bike at home that I use when it's into the minus twenty or colder range outside. Biking isolates the leg muscles and avoids that entire pavement-pounding problem of jogging."

"I don't know. I feel so out of shape, I'm not even sure where to start."

"*Today* was your start," I countered. "The challenge now is to fit a walk in tomorrow, and every day thereafter. I'll give you a prescription to help get you on the right track."

"What, another drug?" she asked with surprise.

"No, better than a drug," I answered. "You're on the deconditioned side of fitness. The only way to improve your exercise capacity is to do more of it. So, let me give you an *exercise* prescription."

"That sounds harder to swallow than a pill," Marion said sarcastically, as she patted her brow with a towel.

"Well, based on today's test, your maximum heart rate was 154 beats per minute. So, a good heart rate zone to work towards during your exercise sessions would be 70 to 85 percent of that," I said, plugging her numbers into my calculator, "or in the range of 110 to130 beats per minute." I handed her a walking exercise prescription (fig. 5.3).

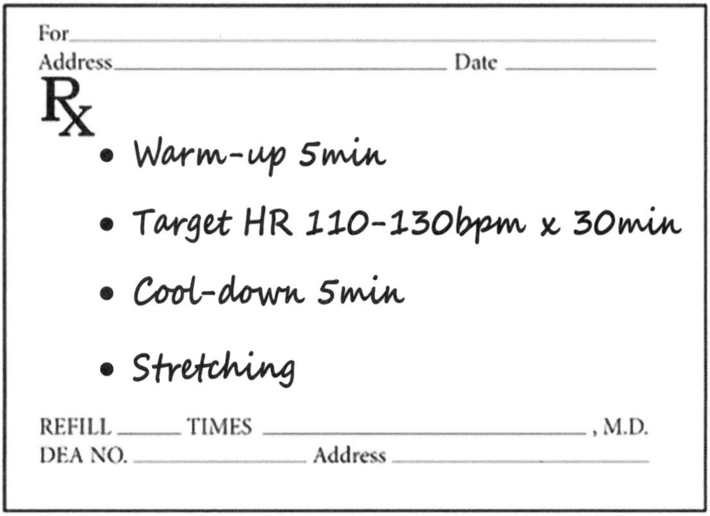

For_____

Address_____ Date _____

Rx

- Warm-up 5min

- Target HR 110-130bpm x 30min

- Cool-down 5min

- Stretching

REFILL _____ TIMES _____ , M.D.

DEA NO. _____ Address _____

Figure 5.3 Walking Exercise Prescription

"Ideally, you'd have your heart rate in this pace target zone for 20 to 30 minutes, but you can work up to this by walking faster for brief periods, say one minute by your watch. Then, you can slow down again to your regular walking speed. You can do two or three of these faster intervals during your first week of regular walking, and then add in more as the weeks go by. This way, you gently expose your body to higher intensity levels of exercise, allowing for ample recovery, and a steady improvement in fitness. It's more fun, too."

"Do I have to exercise with a heart rate monitor?" Marion asked.

"It can be helpful. When you're beginning an exercise program, a heart rate monitor can give you an idea of what moderate-intensity exertion feels like. I rented a heart rate monitor from the local Running Room for a couple of weeks when I was starting my marathon training. Alternatively, the 'talk test' is a pretty reliable way of checking to see if you're in the right exercise zone."

"Oh? What's the talk test?" she asked as she finished her water.

"The talk test is simple: if you can talk, you're exercising in the right zone. Walking fast enough so you break a sweat but can still speak in sentences correlates well with the moderate-intensity exercise zone of a heart rate in the 70 to 85 percent range. By contrast, if you're sauntering along and able to sing *Carefree Highway* by Gordon Lightfoot, then your heart rate is likely under the 70 percent mark, and you need to step things up. On the other extreme, if you're walking so fast that you can't speak in sentences at all, you've probably entered the high-intensity zone and should ease up a notch," I explained.

"People will think I'm crazy if I'm walking around the neighbourhood talking to myself," Marion laughed.

"Not these days," I countered. "With everyone on their Bluetooth, people will just figure you're on a call. Besides, it's probably best to exercise with others. We benefit from being in a community on a variety of fronts, furthering our fitness level included. You'll have more success with motivation and more fun during the exercise activity if you team up with other people and chat while you exercise. The YMCA has a variety of exercise programs you could consider taking that are wonderfully social and the Walking Room is a very supportive venue for those just beginning. A Lone Ranger-styled exercise program tends to be lonely, limited in vista, frustrating, and more readily discarded. Better is a group approach to regular exercise with the 'All for one, and one for all' *Three Musketeers*' motto," I said. "So, for starters, why don't you take your husband, Bill, out for a walk? He could also benefit from some daily exercise."

The Good Fight

Neil Armstrong may have believed that "every human has a finite number of heartbeats," and he may have even used that idea as an excuse not to "waste any of mine running around doing exercises." But, come on now, "Earth to Neil, hello?! This is ground control to Major Tom... can you hear me, Major Tom?" In the face of our current scientific understanding regarding the enormous health benefits of exercise, this sort of thinking truly belongs on the moon. Even for those people who abuse their bodies with fatty foods, cigarettes, and hours on Playstation-3, more often than not, the heart still amazingly takes a licking and keeps on ticking. President John F. Kennedy more accurately nailed the concern over sedentary living when he wisely said, "We are under-exercised as a nation. We look instead of play. We ride instead of walk. Our existence deprives us of the minimum physical activity essential for healthy living." Sedentary behaviour is not only an established risk factor for developing heart disease and stroke; it is the paramount reason for our current epidemics of diabetes, high blood pressure, and obesity. If we are interested in reducing our vascular risk and making some headway on the weight maintenance front, we need to get out from behind our computer monitors and take part in daily exercise. Otherwise, sitting and staying *logged on* might accelerate our final *log out*.

We need to rethink the value of regular exercise. As a standalone weight-loss strategy, exercise may not completely return our bodies to their svelte teenage shapes, but the health benefits of exercise are several and substantial, the majority of which are well within the reach of most people taking part in moderately intense exercises and activities. In fact, the largest benefits come when sedentary folk get off the couch and burn as little as 800 to 1200 calories per week, or the equivalent of about thirty minutes of brisk walking per day.[94] While there are more fitness gains to be had with longer and more intense exertion, the relationship between expected health benefits and the amount of weekly exercise isn't a linear one (fig. 5.4).[95] Exercise-related health benefits begin to level off at higher levels of physical exertion. This means that the incremental benefits of exercising wane as we move from walker to runner or from participant to athlete. That's not to say we shouldn't aspire to become runners or athletes, but it does say that we need to at least become participants and walk.

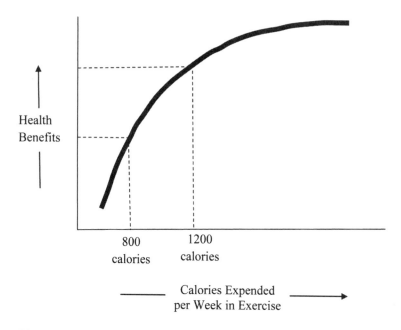

Fig. 5.4 Increasing Health Benefits with Increasing Amounts of Exercise

Marrying healthy dietary choices to a regular exercise program is not only the quintessential way to reduce abdominal fat, it is the central means for protecting our cardiovascular system from disease. More important than mirror appeal are the numerous ways that exercise fights against the risk factors that make up the metabolic syndrome. Specifically, regular exercise can help counter high blood pressure,[96] abnormal blood sugar and insulin levels,[97] as well as off-kilter blood cholesterol and triglyceride levels (fig. 5.5).[98] Exercise may not be the only way to counteract the metabolic syndrome; it just happens to be the healthiest and most cost effective way.

F	Fat Reduction
I	Improved Blood Pressure
G	Glucose Stabilization
H	HDL Enhancement
T	Triglyceride Reduction

Table 5.1 How Exercise Fights the Metabolic Syndrome

In the Swedish Obesity Study, it's been shown that bariatric surgery can offset the abnormalities of the metabolic syndrome and reduce mortality rates in those patients who are severely obese.[99] This is wonderful news. Up until recently, palliative care was pretty much all I had to offer my morbidly obese patients. They would roll into my office on their motorized scooters, too heavy to walk, with legs swollen beyond recognition and, after reviewing their medications, I would encourage them as best I could to "try and carry on," knowing full well that the carrying on wouldn't be for much longer. So, I'm delighted to offer select patients the proven effective rescue of bariatric surgery. However, these data in no way diminish the importance of exercise. After recovery from their life-saving surgery, it is imperative that these patients join the gym to manage their weight and establish cardiovascular health.

Raise a Little HDL

One of the beneficial mechanisms of exercise is its ability to protect our blood vessels from cholesterol build-up. Each and every one of us have floating in our circulation a fleet of proteins known as High Density Lipoproteins, or HDLs; these remove cholesterol from our blood vessels and can reduce the size of our vascular plaques. Regular exercise increases our "good" HDL-C levels and helps to reduce the "bad" Low Density Lipoprotein cholesterol levels (LDL-C).[100] HDL works by reversing the flow of cholesterol away from our blood vessels and decreasing the amount in our blood vessel walls (fig. 5.5).

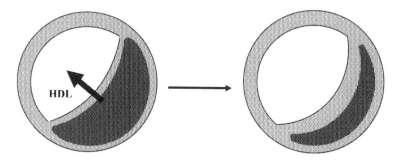

Fig. 5.5 HDL Removes Cholesterol from Blood Vessels

HDL binds onto the cholesterol it finds messing with our heart, including the cholesterol sitting within the walls of our blood vessels, and shuttles it back to our livers in a process called the reverse transport mechanism. From there, the cholesterol, which is a key heart attack inducing ingredient, gets processed into something more useful for our body, like growth hormone for muscle building, or it gets added to our bile and makes its way south to visit the Tidy Bowl man. Each HDL steadily grows in size as it makes its pilgrimage from peripheral tissue to liver, reducing harmful cholesterol levels and our risk of vascular trouble as it goes.[101]

We can assess the extent of our reverse cholesterol transport by measuring the amount of HDL bound to cholesterol in our blood, called the HDL-cholesterol level (HDL-C). When it comes to predicting heart attack risk, HDL-C is like a crystal ball. The Framingham study showed that the risk of developing heart disease varied considerably, depending upon the HDL-C.[102] Those patients who had the lowest HDL-C levels had ten times the risk of dying of a heart attack, compared with those who had the highest HDL-C levels. Fortunately, HDL-C levels aren't carved in stone. With some attention to regular exercise, it's possible to increase our HDL-C levels, no matter where they may currently sit, and to stabilize our cholesterol plaques, no matter where they're currently sitting.

Unfortunately, the HDL-driven reverse transport system can get quickly overwhelmed by the lipid-laden lives we lead, where cholesterol is continually pushed forward from our plates into our blood vessels. So, for optimal improvements in raising our HDL-C levels and reducing our LDL-C levels, we need to give some thought to improving the health of our diets, as well as to increasing the time spent in our walking shoes. Some might argue that all of these lifestyle approaches are too hard won for their minimal HDL-C raising effects; however, it's important to bear in mind that even small changes in HDL-C levels can have dramatic benefits for heart health. For every one percent rise in HDL-C, the risk of having a heart attack drops by a corresponding one percent.[103] If we want to reduce the risk of heart attack and stroke, it's critical to reverse the flow of cholesterol away from our blood vessels. Even baby steps, taken in the right direction, will move us a long way on the road of health.

Survival of the Fittest

In terms of longevity, many factors, including genetic giftedness and luck of the draw might help explain why some people make it into the centenarian club while others succumb to premature illness. But one key reason that consistently rises to the top of the heap is survival of the fittest, or, more specifically, survival because of fitness. By the term fitness, I'm not referring to Charles Darwin's controversial evolutionary theory and the so-called natural selection of butterflies and baboons, but rather to demonstrable cardiorespiratory fitness, clearly defined as how efficiently our bodies can make use of the air we breathe. The more oxygen our exercising muscles can grab hold of, the more fit we are. It's a complicated bit of physiology involving not only the ability of our heart and lungs to convey oxygen to our exercising muscles but of the ability of our muscles themselves—and their metabolic machinery—to make use of the oxygen that comes their way. Power, strength, speed, and endurance all depend upon how efficient our muscle cells are in taking up oxygen from the circulating red blood cells, so that energy stored in the form of sugar and fat molecules can be converted into usable work energy. Athletes have extensive metabolic machinery that proficiently does this; folks who live their lives from an armchair do not.

Cardiorespiratory fitness is the single most important independent predictor of longevity; even more important than the amount of excess body weight we're carrying around. Dr. Steven Blair, from the Cooper Institute in Texas, demonstrated this by testing fitness levels in a large group of adults and then following them over time. He found that the level of fitness maintained by each of his subjects was the most important predictor for survival.[104] In particular, he noticed that the overweight people in his study who demonstrated a moderate level of fitness had a significantly lower risk of heart disease than did the thin, but sedentary individuals.[105] Likewise, irrespective of body weight, physical fitness was found to substantially reduce the risk of stroke (fig. 5.6).[106] No matter what body habitus you were dealt, fitness trumps fatness every time.

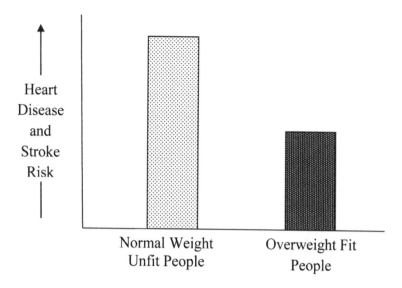

Fig. 5.6 Fitness Trumps Fatness

The gold standard for defining cardiorespiratory fitness is a parameter called VO_2max, which is a measure of our bodies' maximum capacity to transport and utilize oxygen. Unlike Churchill's V for victory, in pulmonary physiology, V represents volume of oxygen, expressed either in litres per minute, or millilitres per kilogram of bodyweight per minute. My VO_2max was measured when I was trying to improve my running time, so I could qualify for the Boston Marathon. I was not only hooked up to electrodes to monitor my heart rate and rhythm (as Marion experienced during her stress test), but I also had to exercise while wearing a face mask. This Darth Vader-like breathing contraption was fit snuggly over my face so that the amount of oxygen I inhaled and the amount of carbon dioxide I exhaled could be accurately measured. The procedure wasn't just a brisk walk, either. I had to run on the treadmill at full tilt, while a couple of exercise technicians in their early twenties egged me on to exhaustion. "Pretty good for an old guy," one tech muttered, as I turned purple with exhaustion and waved them to stop. But since directly measuring VO_2max is too cumbersome for day-to-day clinical medicine, we estimate the fitness levels of our patients using a treadmill or stationary bicycle testing, without all the breathing machinery. It's close enough for practical purposes and allows us to quite easily follow their progress over time. There are even simpler tests that also predict fitness levels with reasonable accuracy, including the Six Minute Walk Test and the Long Corridor Walk Distance.[107] Although tall, lean, young men typically do the best at these tests, walking with their long easy strides, all of us should be able to make it around a 400-meter track (quarter-mile) in less than six minutes. This is important, since studies have shown that the risk of death increases if you can't, especially if your six minute walk test distance is less than 350 meters.[108]

Although our fitness level (VO_2max) is dependent on body size, gender, age, and genetics, it can be improved with exercise training.[109] The good news is that you don't have to be a born athlete or a dedicated fitness fanatic from the 80s, complete with cotton sweatband and matching leg warmers, to do so. Research has confirmed that those who adopt a physically active lifestyle—even as late as middle age and beyond—can still enjoy a reduction in mortality that's similar to those who have been physically active throughout their whole lives. It's never too late to make exercise a regular part of your day.[110] And it's not as if you have to train to be an Olympian to improve your longevity. In addition to your absolute fitness level, an important determinant of long term survival is the amount of fitness improvement you achieve.[111] This is particularly the case for those who move from a sedentary lifestyle to a more active one. It's a bit like getting an A for effort in grade school, even though you didn't make the honor roll. So, who cares if you can't jog a mile without stopping to pretend to tie your shoelaces; the more you work at improving your fitness level, the greater will be your health reward. There's no time to lose. You can begin to improve your VO_2max today, even during your next walk. All you need to do is pick up the pace a bit, and not necessarily for the entire walk, but just for a certain distance, such as to the next light standard, or the fire hydrant at the corner. Then, you can slow down again to your regular walking pace, and catch your breath while you prepare for the next brisker walking segment. Brief pulses of more intense exercise is a sure-fire way of developing our VO2max.[112] In the running world, this method of training is referred to 'Fartlek', which is Swedish for 'speed play.' It was developed back in the 1930s by former Olympian, Gustaf Holmér and proved successful for his cross-country running team. Incorporating short periods of higher-intensity exercise into our activities and workouts is a safe way of telling our bodies to build up the oxygen utilization machinery within our muscle cells.

It's a gentle form of interval training that not only effectively improves aerobic fitness levels, but also efficiently burns fat, and makes the trek around the neighborhood a lot more enjoyable.

Fat Burning Zone?

"But hey, what about the 'fat-burning zone?' Isn't doing long, low-intensity workouts, like two hours on the elliptical or three on the Stairmaster the best way to burn fat?" some might argue. Well-ingrained into our modern fitness mindset is the assertion that low-intensity exercise (defined by an exercising heart rate in the range of 40 to 60 percent of a person's maximal heart rate, or MHR) consumes a higher percentage of energy from fat, as opposed to high-intensity exercise (defined by a heart rate response greater than 85 percent of the maximal heart rate, or MHR), which consumes a higher percentage of energy from glycogen (the ready-to-use storage form of carbohydrate found in muscle and liver cells). Table 5.2 shows the fat to glycogen ratios and that lower-intensity walking exercise burns proportionally more fat than higher-intensity running exercise.

Fuel Source	Walking (40-60 % MHR)	Running (> 85% MHR)
Fat Stores	40%	25%
Glycogen Stores	60%	75%

Table 5.2 Exercise Intensity and Ratio of Fuel Sources

However, this type of thinking is misleading. Sure, when the body needs energy in a slow and steady manner, such as sitting here reading this book or walking in the park, the ratio of fat consumption to glycogen utilization may be higher. Likewise, during more intense activities, such as when you miss the first bus and you have to bust your Beatle boots to catch *the one after 909,* the ratio of glycogen consumption to fat would likely be higher, so the body can meet its more immediate energy needs. But these numbers represent ratios, not calories. If you want to lose weight in the form of excess fat, it's calories you need to burn, not mathematical quotients. It's less important *where* the energy is derived and more important *how much* energy is consumed. For example, after thirty minutes of exercise, a seventy kilogram person will burn far more calories while running than while walking—some 300 calories more (table 5.3). So, whether the proportion of energy derives more from glycogen stores or from fat stores isn't really the concern; the higher the intensity of the exercise, the greater the fat burn because the overall number of calories burned is higher.[113]

Fuel Source Calories	Walking (lower intensity)	Running (higher intensity)
Fat Calories	52 kcal	107 kcal
Glycogen Calories	78 kcal	430 kcal
Total calories	130 kcal	430 kcal

Table 5.3 Exercise Intensity and Calorie Consumption

There's no question that exercising for long periods of

time will burn calories, including those derived from fat. But, few of us have unlimited hours to devote to exercise. The best that I can typically do is forty-five to sixty minutes of exercise per day. Besides, even if I had more protected time to work out, I'd still want to make my exercise sessions as efficient as possible. Why stare at a blank wall, or worse, binge-watch *Game of Thrones*, while pedaling on your stationary bike in your unfinished basement any longer than absolutely necessary? It may be helpful to consider what comprises the calorie-burning equation:

$$Cal = Wt \times time \times intensty$$

Calories burned during exercise =
Bodyweight x Exercise Duration x Exercise Intensity

This means that a heavy person walking for a long time will obviously burn more calories than a light person walking for a shorter duration. But if time is limited, regardless of your weight, more calories will be expended in a shorter time, at higher exercise intensities. What's more, when the workout is over and the après exercise snacks abound, higher intensity exercise continues to provide dividends. Exercising hard liberates more fatty acids into our circulation and more effectively quells our appetite. As well, if we do decide to eat following a higher intensity workout (such as a stationary bicycle spin class), fewer consumed calories get converted into fat than following lower intensity activities (such as reading *Vogue* on a stationary bicycle with a pedal revolution speed of three per minute).[114] Health gains don't necessarily require us to experience pain, but if we want to improve our fitness levels and have more success with our weight-control efforts, we should consider ramping it up a notch.

Rush Hour, Too

"Who can afford the time to exercise every day?" my patients often ask after I give them my exercise pitch. And it's a reasonable question. On hectic days, when consultation requests from the emergency room add to my morning workload forcing my clinic to run through lunch, or when the burgeoning business agenda extends our staff meetings into the evening, my hallowed exercise time gets sacrificed to the jealous god of hustle and bustle, too. But in light of the manifold health benefits of exercise, including its central role in weight management, my question is this: "Who can afford *not* to exercise?" With the prevalence of diabetes, high blood pressure, and obesity skyrocketing out of control, nobody can afford to miss a day's exercise. As cartoonist Randy Glasbergen joked, "What fits your busy schedule better, exercising one hour a day or being dead 24-hours a day?"

We need to be flexible and creatively search out potential opportunities to add some exercise into our day: like a morning walk before work, a swim before dinner, or an evening stroll. How about this? Rather than driving your car all over town, take your bicycle out for a spin instead? In Bogota, Colombia, bike-friendly urban planning has encouraged cycling as a major transportation mode, resulting in improved air quality for the city and improved quality of life for its citizens.[115] Although the infrastructure of North American cities seems more designed for car travel, we'll have more success with weight control if we can shift our mode of transportation from passive car driving to active walking or bicycling. A survey in Atlanta, Georgia found that for each additional hour commuters spent driving their cars per day, there was a 6 percent increase in the risk of developing obesity.[116] No matter how busy our lives may feel, we can't afford this kind of risk-laden time. Even replacing our shortest car trips—the ones in the two to three mile range, for example—with walking or cycling, would allow most of us to achieve the physical activity levels needed for cardiovascular health maintenance and weight control. I have recently made a concerted effort to bike to the hospital during the spring and summer months. With the snail-paced traffic congestion through Edmonton's downtown, it takes me no longer to bike to work and the benefits are substantial: I fit in two workouts, I feel energized for the day, and I don't produce any unnecessary greenhouse gases for the environment. Active transport in the form of walking or cycling offers the greatest potential to not only reduce air pollution but to reduce our cardiovascular risk factors and our waist circumference. The Heart and Stroke slogan,

"Ride for Heart," pegs the solution squarely. So, let's think globally and ride locally.

Champ at the Bit

When I joined our school's cross-country running club, Jim Fixx was a running icon. He was partially responsible for igniting the fitness fixation that swept North America in the 1970s. His road to health was an inspiring story. His father had died of a heart attack at the age of forty-three and, determined not to follow those fatal footsteps, he quit smoking, took up regular jogging, and shed some fifty pounds of excess belly baggage. For Fixx, jogging then led to running, and this became his vehicle to fame and fitness. As detailed in his 1977 best-selling publication *The Complete Book of Running*, he knew a great deal about how to maximize the benefits of endurance exercise. However, what he didn't know, or at least what he chose not to learn, was that he himself had significant atherosclerotic plaque buildup on his heart arteries. Genetic predisposition has this ugly way of raining on the best of parades. He had elevated cholesterol and, supposedly, even symptoms of chest pain when he exercised. Despite being urged to undergo stress testing by Dr. Cooper, of the renowned Cooper Institute in Texas, he ignored medical advice and continued to train vigorously. Unfortunately, as beneficial as exercise is for heart health, it isn't a standalone strategy. While jogging at the age of fifty-two years, he died of a heart attack, thereby tainting his proud running legacy with concerns of safety about the sport.

While those who exercise may be at a slightly increased risk during the hour or so of training—particularly during a stressful event like a marathon or a triathlon competition—for the remainder of the day, their risk of heart trouble, including sudden death, is significantly lower than that of the couch potatoes in the crowd and can actually extend their longevity substantially. However, a healthy dose of caution remains advisable; we need to take care. When I discuss the benefits of exercise with my sedentary patients in clinic (which seems to be pretty much every patient I see these days), I review five proven-effective means of reducing the risk of exercise-related troubles. For ease of memory, I've fashioned them into the acronym CHAMP, detailed as follows (table 5.4).

Check-up	Get your doctor's blessing
Habitual	Exercise most days
Avoid Extremes	Avoid hot and cold temperatures
Moderate Intensity	Follow the talk test
Pre and post Precautions	Always warm up and cool down

Table 5.4 Reducing the Risks of Exercise

Check-up

All workout equipment and exercise programs have medical disclaimers set out in bold print suggesting that clients "seek medical advice before using." Such stipulations are a good idea because we are unique individuals, each with specific health needs and medical issues. So, to minimize injury during exercise, everyone can benefit from customized, professional advice. The family physician, with ready access to your medical history, is the ideal person to start with. Begin your exercise program by touching base with your doctor; they'll be delighted to hear of your interest and will be able to speak to any concerns you might have about your specific risk of exercising. The American College of Sports Medicine recommends that patients at risk for heart artery disease undergo symptom-limited stress testing prior to embarking on a strenuous exercise program.[117] Exercise stress testing is by no means a guarantee that heart trouble won't come knocking on your door, but it's a simple doctor-supervised screening tool that provides a current snapshot of your exercise capacity and can uncover treatable problems such as blood flow abnormalities and heart rhythm disturbances, as well as help predict who is at increased risk for future cardiovascular calamity.[118]

Habitual

Even though a single bout of exercise has been shown

to significantly improve cardiovascular parameters, like insulin sensitivity, for example,[119] health benefits are compounded with the more we do. Sporadic exertion doesn't provide the same health benefits as regular exercise and exposes the weekend warrior to musculoskeletal injury and cardiovascular risk. Unfortunately, the benefits of exercise can't be stored up for a rainy day. Exercise, much like taking a blood pressure medication, is most cardioprotective when attended to on a daily basis.[120] Having been on the high school football team may be a nice memory, but when it comes to your present fitness level, it's joined the ranks of your dusty grad photo and 70s vinyl collection and is long forgotten by your heart and blood vessels. Exercise is easiest to remember, and most enjoyable, when it becomes a regular part of your routine. Recognizing that there may be times when exercise just isn't feasible, we need to creatively consider how we can fit some form of physical exercise into most days of our week. Ideally, exercise should be a daily habit, like brushing your teeth, making your bed, and eating your veggies. And, it's one habit you'll never have to break.

Avoid extremes

Time of day, ambient temperature, and duration of exercise all play into the potential risks of exertion. As we know, the stress hormone cortisol peaks in the early morning hours; so, our blood vessels don't need us adding physical stress to the already stressful morning mix. It is one thing for an experienced athlete to do training in the early morning hours, but quite another for a previously sedentary person to embark on a 6 a.m. hill-sprinting session. Better to take a walk around the park with Fido in the early morning air and wake up the body more gently. Likewise, exercising late in the evening, particularly at night, presents certain dangers, not the least of which is getting struck by a car while jogging across a poorly lit intersection. A workout session before bed can also make it more difficult to relax and may interfere with sleep onset. So, exercising somewhere in the middle of the day is probably best, when your body is awake and you have no immediate plans to sleep.

In terms of ambient temperature, it's best to avoid exercising in really hot or cold temperatures. I don't think that you should just sit on the couch on those days, but you should consider exercising inside, instead, such as on a treadmill or stationary bike in your basement. High temperatures cause blood vessels to dilate, reducing exercise efficiency and exposing you to fluid and electrolyte disturbances, and the possibility of heat exhaustion and heatstroke. Cold temperatures are also trouble because they make blood vessels constrict, or narrow, potentially reducing blood flow to the heart muscle. If there are narrowed plaques already present in your heart's blood vessels, then heart trouble can follow. This is why heart attack rates typically increase after a snowfall when otherwise sedentary folks take to shoveling their driveways.[121]

Too long an exercise session can increase the risk of

musculoskeletal injury, as well as fluid and electrolyte imbalances, and vascular stress. After about an hour of intense exercise, cortisol levels increase and counteract the muscle-building process, putting a cap on the further benefits of ongoing exercise.[122] Keeping the workout to under an hour, or breaking up the exercise session into two or three shorter sessions, can get around this. It's useful to know that exercise time is additive. A fifteen-minute walk in the morning, plus twenty-five minutes on the stationary bike over the lunch hour, and then a twenty-minute walk before dinner, all add up to sixty minutes of exercise in total—an ideal amount for the day.

Moderate intensity

The adage "all things in moderation" may not apply to body piercing or glue sniffing, but in reference to exercise, it is wisdom that's bang on. While high-intensity training is necessary to achieve Olympic gold, it's unnecessary for cardiovascular health, and certainly not without potential danger. By contrast, moderate-intensity exercise maximizes the benefits of exercise and minimizes the risks. One way to define exercise intensity is by measuring heart rate. When your exercising heart rate enters the range of 70 to 85 percent of your maximal heart rate (MHR), you've arrived in the moderate zone. (Maximal heart rate can be estimated using the simplified formula: 220 minus your age). Getting hold of a heart rate monitor can make this determination all the easier. Alternatively, you can estimate moderate intensity exertion by your ability to speak in sentences while you exercise. If you're able to make conversation and still break a sweat, then perfect, you're in the moderate-intensity zone. If, however, you're panting so hard during your workout that you sound like a telegraph report, you're probably working too hard and should ease up a little. Conversely, if you can sing The Hallelujah chorus from Handel's *Messiah* or recite Shakespeare's "What light through yonder window breaks?" soliloquy while exercising, quit with the drama and increase the intensity of your workout. When we exercise in this moderate zone we stimulate our cellular machinery to more efficiently make use of oxygen. After as little as two to three weeks of daily, thirty-minute, moderately-intense workouts, fitness levels will measurably improve. In no other pursuit can mediocrity provide such life-saving results as this. These noticeable fitness improvements can often act as an important source of motivation. This is especially the case if a log is kept, recording some of the work-out details—a technique used routinely by elite athletes. There's nothing like a PB (Personal Best) to spur one's commitment to keep going, higher, faster, stronger.

Pre and Post Exercise Precautions

Bookending our work-outs with some intentional easy-does-it activity can help to reduce the risk of exercise. As outlined in the walking prescription below (table 5.5), three to five minutes at the beginning and end of our exercise time should be set aside for health's sake. The heart doesn't like abrupt starts and stops. Just like saying "Hey Honey, wake up," isn't sufficient foreplay; so, too, we need to adequately prepare our bodies for exercise. But, unlike intimate relations, five minutes by the clock is all that's required to warm up before entering into a workout session. The pre-exercise warm-up is recommended primarily to protect muscles from injury. Those who save time and skip the warm-up session often pay big time with soft tissue injuries and set themselves backwards on the road to improved fitness rather than forwards. The warm-up period can also provide important feedback about whether exercise is a good idea. Sometimes, it can be difficult to differentiate *blah* feelings from being under the weather with the early symptoms of a cold or the flu. When I'm not sure, I use the warm-up period to provide the answer. If I feel improved after warming up, I go for the gusto. However, if I continue to feel poorly, I give exercise a miss for the day. We shouldn't exercise if we're not feeling well. There's no advantage to the body health-wise and there are considerable risks. Listening to our bodies is the most important ingredient in reducing these risks. If Jim Fixx had done this, he might still be alive and well today.

Cooling down after exercise is also important, not so much to prevent muscular injury, but more to allow your heart an opportunity to slow down gently. A mirror image of the warm-up, the cool down helps protect against heart rhythm disturbances or rapid drops in blood pressure. When we stop exercising abruptly, blood return to our heart is reduced, since it's the exercising muscles that pump blood back to our hearts. As a result, if we jump off the treadmill after going full speed, it's not just twisting our ankle that's at stake; our blood pressure can drop precipitously. This is why sprinters always do a victory lap after breaking the finish line tape. Sure, they love the applause, catching roses from the crowd, and wearing their country's flag like a cape, but they also know full well that if they sprint and stop, they'll sprint and drop.

Including some gentle stretching exercises after the warm-up and at the end of the cooldown will speed up muscular recovery from the workout and improve general flexibility. The key muscles to stretch for a walking workout include the hamstrings, calves, and quadriceps. To stretch the hamstring muscles, try leaning forward with outstretched arms onto the back of a chair in front of you, bending at the waist, and keeping your legs straight. For a calf stretch, stand a meter from the wall, lean forward, placing outstretched hands at shoulder width on the wall, as if being frisked by the police. And, to stretch the quadriceps muscles, use a wall for balance, bend one leg at the knee and, holding onto the raised ankle, pull the heel up to your buttocks for a gentle stretch of the front of the thigh muscles. Take your time and don't overstretch. When it comes to stretching, regular, gentle, and slow is the best combination for success.

Warm Up	Walk for 3-5 minutes at easy talking pace to warm leg muscles. Warm-up target heart rate zone: 60-70 percent of maximum heart rate. Stretch hamstrings, calves, and quadriceps muscles before commencing pace workout
Pace	Walk briskly with intention for 30 minutes. Break a sweat but still be able to talk, not sing. Target heart rate zone: 70-85 percent of maximum heart rate. Option of interspersing 1-2 minutes of easy walking every 10 minutes until conditioned.
Cool Down	Walk easily for 3-5 minutes at comfortable talking pace again, to slow heart rate After you stop, heart rate should drop by over 12 bpm after first minute of rest and over 22 bpm after two minutes of rest. Stretch hamstrings, calves and quadriceps muscles

Table 5.5 Walking Exercise Prescription

Fitness Burns Fatness

"All fine and good with aerobic fitness," you say, but your real interest right now is getting rid of the excess fat from around your midriff. Well, covering your body with "detoxifying" Saran Wrap won't help, nor will wearing heated "slenderizing" jeans, or hooking yourself up to some *I Love Lucy*-style body jiggler. If you're serious about slimming down, forget the gadgets and gimmicks that promise to "melt the fat away," and instead lay your hands on a medicine ball or a pair of dumbbells. Muscle tissue is where fat gets burned; it's that simple. Celebrities know this full well. According to *US Magazine*, Mariah Carey lost her twenty pounds and three sizes through "serious sweat sessions" with her personal trainer, sometimes up to one and a half hours of exercise per day.[123] If there were an easier way to lose fat, then surely the pop idols, dependent upon their body image as their calling cards, would be all over it.

Muscle tissue burns fat in three complementary ways. First, fat gets consumed inside muscle cells while they are actively working, contracting, and relaxing. Muscle cell machinery, consisting of an array of contractile proteins called myofilaments, makes use of fat as fuel. Studies have shown that our muscle tissue preferentially mobilizes and metabolizes fatty acids from adipose tissue during exercise.[124] In other words, muscle eats fat. As muscle cells are stimulated to increase in size, fat is consumed and fat cells shrink in size (fig. 5.7). It follows then, that the bigger the muscles being exercised, the bigger the fat burn. This is why exercises like walking, jogging, and cycling, which make use of the large leg muscle group are more efficient fat-burning activities than ventures like forearm curls, triceps extensions, or finger calisthenics.

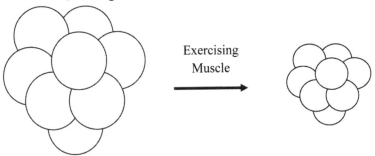

Fig. 5.7 Exercising Muscle Causes Fat Cell Shrinkage

As well, exercises that make use of multiple muscle groups—like swimming, rowing, or cross-country skiing— are also very efficient fat burners. If you prefer to start in the privacy of your own home, many exercises can be done with simple equipment, like a medicine ball and a floor mat. Referred to as functional exercises because they mimic real-life activities, these training techniques involve composite full-body movements and make use of multiple muscle groups, including our core abdominal muscles. Such exercises not only burn fat effectively but also enhance flexibility and balance. Online resources, such as the Nike Training Club (NTC) program, available as a cellphone apps (www.nike.com/ca/ntc-app), can provide expert circuit workouts with clear demonstrations of exercises and tips to achieve your best form. Alternatively, you could enlist the help of a personal trainer at your local recreation facility for a list and demonstration of functional exercises. They can provide detailed, personalized instruction on exercise types and form, so you can get the most benefit out of the activity with the least risk of injury.

Second, muscle cells continue to burn fat after they recover from an exercise session. When we improve our muscular tone by lifting weights (ideally under the expert supervision of a personal trainer), we don't just burn calories during the exercise itself, but long after we've walked home from the gym. Bodybuilders call this phenomenon *the afterburn*. Part of the reason why resistance exercise burns calories even after the exercise has finished is related to muscle repair. Our bodies work on an as-needed basis. For example, when we grab hold of a dumbbell and put our arms to work by slowly flexing our biceps muscle and lifting the weight repeatedly up and down, we tell our bodies that our puny arms are important to us; so, how about giving them a little attention. This muscle loading stimulates a rebuilding process as our body endeavours to improve the strength of our biceps, so they can better meet our weightlifting needs in preparation for a future workout. It takes energy to accomplish this refurbishing process. And, here's the really good news: our bodies obtain that energy from our fat stores and, in particular, from our abdominal fat stores. It's like a double blessing: your arms get stronger and your waistline gets slimmer, all in one go.

To achieve this positive adaptation, we need to provide our exercising muscles with enough load to stimulate the rebuilding process. Based on what's called the *overload principle,* the training stimulus must be greater than what our muscles are accustomed to.[125] Similar to a tailored drug dose, this strength-building dose will need to be individualized—yours will be different than mine, and different from Auntie Jean's. While a personal trainer can be instrumental in individualizing the appropriate weight needed for a particular exercise, in general, the higher the repetitions of an exercise, the lower the amount of weight needed to obtain an adequate muscular stimulus. Bodyweight exercises are an excellent place to start, particularly for those who are new to resistance exercises. They are not only safe to do, but by mimicking our activities of daily living, they improve joint range of motion, and when done in sequence, can provide full-body muscular toning. Compound exercises that make use of multi-joint movements—those that work several muscles or muscle groups at one time—provide the most functional benefits. When we advance to the point of adding weights to our routine, a medicine ball or light dumbbells would be the next step. While it's best to choose a weight that will stimulate our muscles, we don't want to sabotage our efforts by injuring ourselves. There's no shame in using lighter weights. It's always better to choose a lower weight and focus on form, than going big and going home… bent over in pain. As a rule of thumb, our working weight should be half of our maximal lifting capacity. We should be able to complete a set of 8 to 12 repetitions of a particular exercise—comfortably but with some effort. In time, repeating this set two or three times during a workout session, with interposed rest and plenty of fluids, will stimulate the desired physiological adaptions.

Good-bye atrophy; hello strength.

Lastly, muscle burns fat by adding to our lean body tissue, increasing our resting metabolic rate. This is because there is a direct relationship between our muscle mass and our metabolic rate—the bigger the biceps and more powerful the pecs, the higher the basal metabolic rate and the greater the fat combustion, even at rest. In fact, the amount of lean body tissue on our bodies is the single most important factor governing our basal metabolic rate—more important than gender or even age. With the exception of our brain and liver, which together account for about 50 percent of our resting metabolic rate, muscle burns more calories than any other tissues in our body.[126] On average, we burn about ten calories per pound of body weight during a day. But, despite what Shylock might have thought, all pounds of flesh are not the same. For every pound of muscle we have on our frame, we burn in the neighbourhood of fifty calories per day—and that's just to maintain resting muscular tone, and doesn't include the serious energy burn that goes down once our muscles get to work.[127] Taken together—fuel consumption, the afterburn, and improved metabolic rate—are part of the reason why resistance exercise, in the form of bodyweight exercises and weightlifting, is such an efficient means of fat reduction.

Defense from Dependency

It's important to realize that there's more to fitness than

our aerobic capacity. Being physically fit entails having some element of cardiorespiratory reserve, to be sure, but fitness also includes our ability to balance, our flexibility, and our muscular strength. While each of these fitness elements is important, muscular strength arguably tops the list, particularly as we age. In addition to the fat-burning benefit, muscular fitness offers the greatest amount of health benefits, and can even help to offset the rapidity of the aging process. This is because our muscles not only protect our joints, improve bone mineral density, and keep us mobile and functional, they also play a central role in maintaining our metabolic health, including control of blood sugar and cholesterol levels. Elderly patients with diabetes, for example, have been shown to have improved glycemic control and lipid profiles after embarking on regular resistance training.[128] So, it's never too late to incorporate some resistance exercises into the weekly exercise routine.

Unfortunately, muscular strength can be a fleeting thing if we don't make it a priority. It's like expensive real estate—if it's not being used, the body sells it off for more energy-efficient fat storage. After the age of thirty, most of us start losing muscle. This loss occurs in a stepwise fashion with every passing year, averaging between 3-8% of our muscle mass per decade. First, the upper body strength goes, then the back muscles wane, and then before you know it, you're asking for help to open the pickle jar. This atrophying process is accelerated by sedentary behavior, and in particular, by bed rest, a muscle's worst enemy. Studies have shown that bedridden young adults can lose up to 5% of their muscle mass after just two weeks, and those over 70 years can lose a whopping 10%.[129] Talk about fast-tracking it to the Pee-wee Herman look-alike contest! So, although it might not be all that noticeable day by day, this age-related exchange of rippling and chisel for rounding and chub is bound to occur unless intentional steps are taken with resistance exercise to counter the decline.

Muscle loss is not simply a matter of losing the beach body. No, muscular atrophy is far more serious than the mere loss of flex appeal. It's our physical capacity and our longevity that are on the line here. This is because, as we age, we experience reduced cellular renewal, resulting in a progressive accumulation of metabolic waste within our cells. This leads to a nasty process called *apoptosis* (cell death) and over time *sarcopenia* (where *sarco* refers to muscle and *penia* to wasting). Sarcopenia represents a loss of muscle strength and mass in older individuals, which increases their risk of falling and impairs their ability to perform regular day to day activities.[130] In time, this wasting can lead to frailty, disability, and hasten the departure of independence and the arrival of the Grim Reaper. How do you spell nursing home? Well, it begins with 'N' which stands for <u>not strong enough</u>.

There is a direct relationship between musculoskeletal fitness and independent living across our lifespan. As we age, our musculoskeletal fitness—including our strength, endurance, and power—can decline to such a degree, that even a small impairment, such as a short hospital stay for an infection, might result in disability. Many elderly people currently live near or even below the functional threshold for dependence (fig. 5.8). This is a precarious place to be hovering, both from a self-care standpoint and for safety's sake. I see this often in my cardiology consultation practice at our geriatric rehabilitation hospital—case after case of decompensated elderly patients admitted to hospital with a fall or a bout of pneumonia, and now too frail to return home. How they were able to function at home never ceases to amaze me. Though many try to resist the idea of assisted living, the reality of their frail condition often leaves them with little choice. If measures had been established earlier to improve muscular fitness, their debilitating frailty could have been avoided, or at least postponed, to allow for more graceful aging.

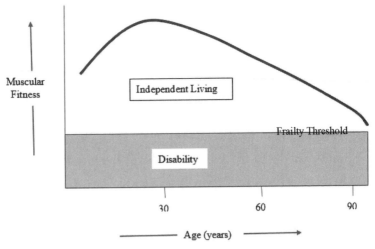

Fig 5.8 Musculoskeletal Fitness and Frailty[131]

The good news is that muscular atrophy can be countered, and if measures are adopted earlier in life, this dismantling process can even be reversed. Although advanced cases of frailty would be the exception, it's usually possible to achieve some level of benefit from routine resistance exercises in most patients. Studies of elderly patients have consistently shown that strength training can significantly improve lean body mass, bone density, and overall fitness level as assessed by peak VO2 determination.[132] Understanding this full well, our geriatric rehab team makes a priority of engaging their elderly patients in daily exercise activities to help counteract sarcopenia and reduce frailty. The point, of course, is not to try to turn grannies into hard bodies, but rather to improve their strength, balance, and coordination, so they can better manage on their own and have an improved quality of life. With this in mind, I underscore the value of strength training with my elderly patients. In those of advanced years, I simplify things by emphasizing the importance of two aspects in particular—hand strengthening and leg strengthening. Both of these are critical for maintaining physical ability— lose them, and lose independent living. To strengthen their hands, I suggest they pick up a gentle handgrip strengthener or some stress balls and use them at least twice a day, such as first thing in the morning and last thing before bed. And, since grip strength can begin to decline as early as the Freedom-55 age, I find myself making similar suggestions to my younger patients, as well. Only, for the younger cohort, I suggest using more heavy-duty strengtheners, like the handgrip crusher. As for leg strengthening, I encourage patients to do body-weight squats. For those of advanced years, I suggest they stand up from their kitchen chair two or three times before each meal. As their leg strength improves, I have them work towards standing from the sitting position without arm assistance. The improvement in their quadriceps muscle strength improves their ability to balance, body transfer, and mobilize without falling. So, while it's never too late to start strength training exercises, there's no time like the present. The earlier we develop a resistance exercise routine, the more meaningful the health gains will be and less the risk of frailty and disability.[133]

Adding Resistance to Marion's Routine

"Do you figure this will help me lose the weight I need to?" Marion asked, as she took my walking exercise prescription and folded it into her purse.

"It certainly won't hurt," I responded, "but losing weight with an exercise program shouldn't be the primary expectation.[134] Exercising muscles burn fat, to be sure, but the lion's share of weight control comes from our diet. Unless you're training for some ironman competition or something, it's just too easy to gain back calories burned during exercise by making bad food choices. Besides, losing weight isn't the only way of achieving a healthier you. Exercise pays health dividends beyond weight control, especially a combination of aerobic and resistance exercises. Have you ever done weights?"

"Weights?" Marion responded with an accompanying facial contortion that provided her answer. "No way. Weights aren't for me!"

"I don't mean Arnold Schwarzenegger bodybuilding," I reassured her with a smile. "I'm talking about muscle toning. Strength is an essential ingredient to whole-body fitness, especially as we age. It helps keep our metabolic risk factors in check, improves our functional abilities, and keeps us living independently for longer."

"But, we don't have any barbells or benches," she argued. "And gyms are far too intimidating. I wouldn't know where to begin."

"Well, a gym membership isn't essential, and you don't need to have a lot of equipment to develop some level of muscular fitness. An exercise mat and medicine ball would be a good place to start, and maybe some light dumbbells in time," I suggested. "During the COVID-19 crisis, when all the gyms were closed, our oldest son got me and my wife onto an online circuit training exercise program that we were able to do at home."

"Well, I'm not very tech-savvy, either," Marion said, shrugging her shoulders.

"That makes two of us, but fortunately it was very easy to access and free to use. Let me show you," I said, pulling up my chair next to hers. "It's this NTC, Nike Training Club app," I said, as I opened the application on my phone.

"There are dozens of expertly-designed workouts from easy beginner options to some challenging high-intensity athletic training, A lot of the workouts take less than ten minutes, like this six-minute *Start-up Benchmark* for example, or this seven-minute *Total-Body Desk Detox.* It's my favorite after my long days sitting and reading echocardiograms."

"I'm not sure," Marion said hesitantly. "I don't have much experience with this sort of thing,"

"Oh, you'll develop that as you go," I said, pointing to my phone's screen, "there's a clear visual demonstration of each exercise you can follow along with, and pleasant verbal cues provided in a charming Kiwi accent to encourage you and keep you using the right form."

"Looks easy enough, I suppose," Marion agreed, as she watched the first exercise demo. "But, I'd rather do walking to build my fitness."

"It's not one or the other," I suggested. "Both stamina and strength are important. Fitness is more than aerobic capacity and walking endurance. As we age, it's vital that we maintain the muscular tone of our body, so we can keep ourselves functional and independent. After all, you don't want to wind up prematurely requiring a nursing home, do you?" I added for rhetorical emphasis.

Marion shook her head and said with surrender, "No, I suppose not. Bill and I love our independence and traveling."

"Well, here's to fitness for life then," I said, as I handed her the NTC app information for downloading. "It'll help you build health, and allow you to enjoy your travels all the more."

Chapter Summary
Fitness Trumps Fatness

- Sedentary behavior is an independent risk factor for developing heart disease and stroke
- Regular exercise stabilizes vascular plaques and reduces the risk of sudden death
- Increasing health benefits come with increasing amounts of exercise with the greatest benefits occurring in previously sedentary folk who take part in regular moderate-intensity activity
- Regular exercise is the most cost-effective way of countering the metabolic syndrome by improving blood pressure, cholesterol and sugar control, and reducing abdominal fat
- Calories burned during exercise = (Bodyweight) x (Duration) x (Intensity)
- Maximal HR = 220 minus Age
- Moderate intensity exercise heart rate zone = 70% to 85% of Maximal HR
- The risk of exercise can be reduced by an adequate warm-up and cool down, avoiding extremes of heat, and exercising in the moderate-intensity zone
- Resistance exercise burns fat in three ways: by

direct consumption, during the rebuilding afterburn process, and by increasing the basal metabolic rate

- The higher the intensity of the exercise, the greater the fat burn
- The four pillars of fitness include cardiorespiratory reserve, balance, flexibility, and muscular strength
- There is a direct relationship between loss of musculoskeletal fitness and frailty
- Hand and quadricep strength are particularly important muscle groups for maintaining independent living

Chapter Notes

84. Fletcher GF, Balady G, Froelicher VF, Hartley LH, Haskell WL, Pollock ML. Exercise standards: a statement for healthcare professionals from the American Heart Association. Special report. Circulation. 1995;91:580-615.

85. Franklin BA, Kahn JK. Delayed progression or regression of coronary atherosclerosis with intensive risk factor modification. Effects of diet, drugs, and exercise. Sports Med. 1996 Nov;22(5):306-20.

86. Wilbert-Lampen U, Leistner D, Greven S, Pohl T, Sper S, Völker C, Güthlin D, Plasse A, Knez A, Küchenhoff H, Steinbeck G. Cardiovascular events during World Cup soccer.N Engl J Med 2008;358 (5):475-83.

87. Hakim AA, Petrovitch H, Burchfiel CM, Ross GW, Rodriguez BL, White LR, Yano K, Curb JD, Abbott RD. Effects of walking on mortality among nonsmoking retired men. N Engl J Med. 1998 Jan 8;338(2):94-9.

88. Manson JE, Hu FB, Rich-Edwards JW, Colditz GA, Stampfer MJ, Willett WC, Speizer FE, Hennekens CH. A prospective study of walking as compared with vigorous exercise in the prevention of coronary heart disease in women.N Engl J Med. 1999 Aug 26;341(9):650-8.

89. Kavanagh T. Exercise in the primary prevention of coronary artery disease. Can J Cardiol 2001;17(2):155-61.

90. Yung LM, Laher I, Yao X, Chen ZY, Huang Y, Leung FP. Exercise, vascular wall and cardiovascular diseases: an update (part 2). Sports Med. 2009;39(1):45-63.

91. Huikuri HV, Castellanos A, Myerburg RJ. Sudden death due to cardiac arrhythmias. N Engl J Med 2001;345(20):1473-82.

92. Ni H, Coady S, Rosamond W, Folsom AR, Chambless L, Russell SD, Sorlie PD. Trends from 1987 to 2004 in sudden death due to coronary heart disease: the Atherosclerosis Risk in Communities (ARIC) study. Am Heart J. 2009 Jan;157(1):46-52.

93. Chugh SS, Reinier K, Teodorescu C, Evanado A, Kehr E, Al Samara M, Mariani R, Gunson K, Jui J. Epidemiology of sudden cardiac death: clinical and research implications. Prog Cardiovasc Dis. 2008 Nov-Dec;51(3):213-28.

94. Exercising Your Post-MI Patient. TK Fenske, M Paletta, B Daub. Patient Care 2001;12(9):85-104.

95. Bouchard C. Physical Inactivity. Can J Cardiol 1999 Dec;Vol 15(Supplement G):89G-92G.

96. Chiong JR. Controlling hypertension from a public health perspective. Int J Cardiol. 2008 Jul 4;127(2):151-6.

97. Healy G, Dunstan D, Salmon J, et al. Objectively measured light-intensity physical activity is independently associated with 2-h plasma glucose. Diabetes Care 2007;30:1384-9.

98. O'Keefe J, Bell D. The post-prandial hyperglycemia/

hyperlipidemia hypothesis: a hidden cardiovascular risk factor? Am J Cardiol 2007;100:899-904.

99. Sjöström L, Narbro K, Sjöström CD, Karason K, Larsson B, Wedel H, Lystig T, Sullivan M, Bouchard C, Carlsson B, Bengtsson C, Dahlgren S, Gummesson A, Jacobson P, Karlsson J, Lindroos AK, Lönroth H, Näslund I, Olbers T, Stenlöf K, Torgerson J, Agren G, Carlsson LM; Swedish Obese Subjects Study. Effects of bariatric surgery on mortality in Swedish obese subjects. N Engl J Med. 2007 Aug 23;357(8):741-52.

100. Tambalis KD, Panagiotakos DB, Kavouras SA, Sidossis LS. Responses of Blood Lipids to Aerobic, Resistance, and Combined Aerobic With Resistance Exercise Training: A Systematic Review of Current Evidence. Angiology. 2008 Oct 30.

101. Kawano M, Shono N, Yoshimura T, Yamaguchi M, Hirano T, Hisatomi A. Improved cardio-respiratory fitness correlates with changes in the number and size of small dense LDL: randomized controlled trial with exercise training and dietary instruction. Intern Med. 2009;48(1):25-32.

102. Wilson PW, D'Agostino RB, Levy D, Belanger AM, Silbershatz H, Kannel WB. Prediction of coronary heart disease using risk factor categories. Circulation. 1998 May 12;97(18):1837-47.

103. Wilson PW, D'Agostino RB, Levy D, Belanger AM, Silbershatz H, Kannel WB. Prediction of coronary heart disease using risk factor categories. Circulation. 1998 May 12;97(18):1837-47.

104. Blair SN, Kampert JB, Kohl HW 3rd, Barlow CE, Macera CA, Paffenbarger RS Jr, Gibbons LW. Influences of cardiorespiratory fitness and other precursors on cardiovascular disease and all-cause mortality in men and women. JAMA. 1996 Jul 17;276 (3):205-10.

105. Timothy S. Church, Yiling J. Cheng, Conrad P. Earnest,

Carolyn E. Barlow, Larry W. Gibbons, Elisa L. Priest and Steven N. Blair. Exercise capacity and body composition as predictors of mortality among men with diabetes. Diabetes Care 27.1 (Jan 2004): p83 (6).

106. Lee CD, Blair SN. Cardiorespiratory fitness and stroke mortality in men. Med Sci Sports Exerc. 2002 Apr;34(4):592-5.

107. Newman AB, Simonsick EM, Naydeck BL, Boudreau RM, Kritchevsky SB, Nevitt MC, Pahor M, Satterfield S, Brach JS, Studenski SA, Harris TB. Association of long-distance corridor walk performance with mortality, cardiovascular disease, mobility limitation, and disability. JAMA. 2006 May 3;295(17):2018-26.

108. Prochaczek F, Winiarska H, Krzyzowska M, Brandt JS, Swida KR, Szczurek ZW, Owczarek A, Galecka J. Six-minute walk test on a special treadmill: Primary results in healthy volunteers. Cardiol J. 2007;14(5):447-52.

109. Shephard RJ. Tests of maximum oxygen intake. A critical review. Sports Med. 1984 Mar-Apr;1(2):99-124.

110. Byberg L, Melhus H, Gedeborg R, et al. Total mortality after changes in leisure time physical activity in 50 year old men: 35 year follow-up of population-based cohort. BMJ March 5, 2009;338:b688.

111. Erikssen G, Liestøl K, Bjørnholt J, Thaulow E, Sandvik L, Erikssen J. Changes in physical fitness and changes in mortality. Lancet 1998; Sep 5;352(9130):759-62.

112. J Appl Physiol. 2015 Sep 15;119(6):753-8.

113. Irving BA, Davis CK, Brock DW, Weltman JY, Swift D, Barrett EJ, Gaesser GA, Weltman A. Effect of Exercise Training Intensity on Abdominal Visceral Fat and Body Composition. Med Sci Sports Exerc. 2008 Oct 8.

114. Yoshioka M, Doucet E, St-Pierre S, Alméras N, Richard D,

Labrie A, Després JP, Bouchard C, Tremblay A. Impact of high-intensity exercise on energy expenditure, lipid oxidation and body fatness. Int J Obes Relat Metab Disord. 2001 Mar;25(3):332-9.

115. Wright L, Fulton L. Climate change mitigation and transport in developing countries. Transport Reviews 2005;25:691-717.

116. Frank LD, Andersen MA, Schmid TL. Obesity relationships with community design, physical activity, and time spent in cars. Am J Prev Med 2004;27:87-96.

117. Yu S, Patterson CC, Yarnell JW. Is vigorous physical activity contraindicated in subjects with coronary heart disease? Evidence from the Caerphilly study. Eur Heart J. 2008 Mar;29(5):602-8.

118. Peterson PN, Magid DJ, Ross C, Ho PM, Rumsfeld JS, Lauer MS, Lyons EE, Smith SS, Masoudi FA. Association of exercise capacity on treadmill with future cardiac events in patients referred for exercise testing. Arch Intern Med. 2008 Jan 28;168(2):174-9.

119. Perseghin G, Price TB, Petersen KF, Roden M, Cline GW, Gerow K, Rothman DL, Shulman GI. Increased glucose transport-phosphorylation and muscle glycogen synthesis after exercise training in insulin-resistant subjects. N Engl J Med. 1996 Oct 31;335 (18):1357-62.

120. Mittleman MA, Maclure M, Tofler GH, et al. Triggering of acute myocardial infarction by heavy physical exertion. N Engl J Med 1993;329:1677-83.

121. Lloyd EL. The role of cold in ischaemic heart disease: a review. Public Health. 1991 May;105(3):205-15.

122. Karkoulias K, Habeos I, Charokopos N, Tsiamita M, Mazarakis A, Pouli A, Spiropoulos K. Hormonal responses to marathon running in non-elite athletes. Eur J Intern Med. 2008 Dec;19(8):598-601.

123. US Weekly April 28,2008 Issue 689;56-61.

124. Stevenson E, Williams C, Mash L, Phillips B, Nute M. Influence of high carbohydrate mixed meals with different glycemic indexes on substrate utilization during subsequent exercise in women. Am J Nutr 2006;84:354-60.

125. Andersen, P., and B. Saltin (1985). Maximal perfusion of skeletal muscle in man. J. Physiol., London 366: 233-249.

126. Holliday MA, Potter D, Jarrah A, and Bearg S. The relation of metabolic rate to body weight and organ size. Pediatric Research 1967;1:185.

127. Grande F. Energetics and weight reduction. Am J Clin Nutr. 1968 Apr;21(4):305-14.

128. Lee J, Kim D, Kim C. Resistance Training for Glycemic Control, Muscular Strength, and Lean Body Mass in Old Type 2 Diabetic Patients: A Meta-Analysis. Diabetes Ther. 2017 Jun;8(3):459-473.

129. Moriera J. et al. Age-dependent effects of bed rest in human skeletal muscle: exercise to the rescue. The Journal of Physiology. January 2016, Volume 594, Issue2.

130. Dhillon R. et al. Pathogenesis and Management of Sarcopenia. Clin Geriatr Med. 2017 Feb; 33(1): 17–26.

131. Adapted from Can J Appl Physiol 2001;26:161-216.

132. Braith et al. Resistance exercise: training adaptations and developing a safe exercise prescription. Heart Fail Rev. 2008;13:69-79.

133. Warburton DE, Gledhill N, Quinney A. The effects of changes in musculoskeletal fitness on health. Can J Appl Physiol 2001;26:161-216.

134. Ross R, Janiszewski PM. Is weight loss the optimal target for obesity-related cardiovascular disease risk reduction? Can J Cardiol. 2008 Sep;24 Suppl D:25D-31D.

Chapter 6
In Defense of Afternoon Snacking
Benefits of Healthy Choices

Marion's "Detox" Delusion

"Can I get your opinion on something?" Marion asked as she rummaged through her large leather handbag. "Our yoga instructor is encouraging everyone in the class to go on this detox diet, but I wanted to check with you first to make sure it's safe for me to do," she said, handing me some stapled pages with the title *Master Cleanse* printed in bold type across the top. "It's going to be a bit of a challenge for me, especially since there's no snacking."

"Hmmmm… looks like a real spring clean for the May Queen," I said, as I rubbed my chin and scanned down the front page. "It says here that the diet involves drinking only lemonade mixed with maple syrup and cayenne pepper. It sounds pretty extreme to me. Are you sure you want to do this?"

"Well, our instructor has some herbal teas that we can drink, too… and it's just for a week," she countered. "Besides, it's supposed to boost our immune function and metabolism, and flush out the waste and toxins that have been making us gain weight in the first place."

"It's a popular idea," I agreed, "that we're accumulating poisons in our body, like pesticides, heavy metals, hormones, and the like. It's appealing to think that we can get rid of them by following a detoxification diet or drinking herbal teas. However, there's no scientific basis to support those assertions."

"But, I see detox diets advertised in the newspaper and by celebrities, like Beyoncé, all the time. I just assumed it was an accepted practice," Marion said with a surprised tone.

"It's an accepted big business, is what it is," I stated emphatically. "And while newspaper columnists should know better than to promote anecdotal information, celebrity icons are not typically known for their critical thinking abilities. Popular diet gurus make exaggerated claims about the merits of detox diets, like improved immune function for example, but little is said about which toxins are supposedly causing us such harm, or, for that matter, how they can be measured in our tissues. These so-called "toxins" are blamed for our decreasing energy levels and increasing waist circumferences, but they remain elusive, undefined, and unmeasured."

"You mean to say no toxins are harming our bodies?" she asked incredulously.

"Oh, sure, there are plenty of toxins that we're exposed to day in and day out, including cigarette smoke, monosodium glutamate, and trans-fatty acids, to name but a few," I agreed.

"But, the way to protect ourselves from them is by limiting our exposure to them, not by drinking copious amounts of lemon juice. As for the numerous, well-defined breakdown products from food, drink, over-the-counter drugs, and prescription medications—such as alcohol, ammonia and urea—our bodies have been designed with numerous elegant and sophisticated mechanisms to deal with them. The liver and kidneys are dedicated to filtering and cleaning our blood and tissues, night and day," I said. "So, the suggestion that we can do the job ourselves by following a simple liquid fast is quite an arrogant claim, and there's no evidence to show that toxins can be eliminated in this way."

"But, I know several people from my yoga class who follow the detox regimen twice a year, and they swear by it," Marion argued. "They lose weight each time and feel invigorated."

"I'm not surprised," I said. "Limiting the week's caloric intake to sweetened lemon juice is bound to produce weight loss. But that weight won't necessarily be fat loss," I cautioned. "Extreme caloric restriction, especially when protein is eliminated, can lead to a loss of muscle mass, which if anything, is going to slow down your metabolism, not speed it up. As for feeling invigorated, it's probably the absence of rich heavy foods, rather than the liquid fast, per se."

"So, you don't see any benefits in following a detox diet, then?" she asked disappointedly.

"Not really. Our bodies aren't like cars that need a biannual oil change. Liquid fasting can potentially do more harm than good. For optimal health, our bodies require a continual provision of vitamins and nutrients incorporated into our day-to-day routine. But, that being said," I conceded, "there may be some profit from a period of disciplined caloric intake—getting us out of a dietary rut, breaking a bad cycle of eating junk food, or going "cold turkey" on food addiction, for example. One of the benefits of following any diet is how it affects our food choices in the longer term. After pushing through an entire week of imbibing little more than sugar water, I'm sure it's true that dieters will more likely crave a piece of fresh fruit over a bag of Cheezies and a pop."

"Yes," Marion nodded, "and as I said, there's absolutely no junk food or snacking for the entire week."

"I'm all in favour of the junk food ban," I said. "But, I don't consider junk food and snacking synonymous. Healthy snacking—that is, small and scheduled nutritional breaks, particularly in the afternoon—can go a long way in aiding weight loss efforts and promoting cardiovascular health."

Food Deprivation Dilemma

One of the important shortcomings of detox diets as a form of weight reduction is that they don't teach proper eating behaviour patterns to help sustain the slimmer, post-detox "new you." Imbibing only cucumber water infused with lemon and cinnamon for weeks on end doesn't teach us how to set aside time for breakfast, or plan and pack a healthy lunch, or how to practice portion control, develop restraint at the all-you-can-eat buffet, or expand our repertoire of healthy snack choices. The same old ideas about food persist and the same old unhealthy eating habits remain, stealthily lurking in the cookie cupboard and waiting to pounce once our fast is broken. As a result, individuals who choose periods of food deprivation as a weight control method are apt to regain weight rapidly once they return to the real world of tantalizing temptations at every turn. A refeeding frenzy often results from the heightened attention that tends to get placed on food during times of caloric restriction.

The effects of starvation were examined in detail back in the 1940s. It was during the latter years of the Second World War that intelligence reports were surfacing about the existence of the dark and dreadful Nazi concentration camps and the horrors that were being perpetrated behind their evil walls. It was becoming increasingly clear that millions of people were suffering in famine-like conditions. Little was known at the time about how best to refeed those subjected to starvation. So, to provide some guidance for relief assistance when the war ended, Allied scientists assembled to address the anticipated famine crisis. Doctor Ancel Keys, the physician responsible for the military K-rations, played a central role in these efforts by setting up an experiment dubbed the Minnesota Starvation Study.[135] He planned to investigate both the physiological and psychological effects of extreme calorie restriction on healthy volunteers and to test various refeeding protocols to determine which would be the most effective for mass implementation. He advertised his need for study volunteers among WWII conscientious objectors and received a surprisingly high level of interest from his *Uncle Sam Wants You... to Starve* posters. He was able to narrow down the participant pool to thirty-six emotionally strong and physically healthy men between the ages of twenty-three and thirty-three years. Dr. Keys then had the volunteers follow a strict calorie-reduced diet of approximately1500 calories per day, to simulate the European famine. The intention was for each participant to lose over 25 percent of their initial body weight. The physiological effects were marked. The study was the first to clearly demonstrate how semi-starvation causes heart rate, blood pressure, and body temperature to fall, as well as basal metabolic rate to slow (they noted a remarkable 40 percent drop in BMR from baseline rates). In fact, our current understanding of the physiological effects of starvation still draws heavily from this wartime study. Although the complete report of the study wasn't published until 1950, the renourishment phase of the study added immeasurably to the success of the Allied refeeding programs, instituted as the war ended and freedom finally came to the captives.[136]

In addition, the Minnesota Starvation Study also provided significant insights into the psychological changes that occur during periods of prolonged caloric deprivation. As it turned out, the physical effects of starvation were only part of the hardships endured by the volunteers. As documented during the twenty-four-week calorie restriction phase of the study, the participants uniformly developed fatigue, depressed mood, social withdrawal, sexual disinterest, mental distress, and even hysteria.[137] Review of the participants' diary records showed that the study volunteers had become preoccupied with food. As the weeks of calorie deprivation continued, culinary topics increasingly dominated their thoughts and filled their journal pages. Food became the major topic of their conversations with each other and their meagre meals became the central highlight of their days. In short, food became the center of their universe. After the six-month semi-starvation portion of the study was completed, the volunteers were placed on a refeeding protocol with increasing caloric increments lasting another three months. Their appetites were insatiable. The more food the volunteers were fed, the more food they craved. And when all calorie restrictions were finally removed, the feeding frenzy really began; so much so that the cooks couldn't keep up with them. The starved subjects gorged themselves in an uncontrolled fashion. They ate continually, stopping only to sleep, and consuming more than 5000 calories per day. Not surprisingly, the participants rapidly regained their lost weight. In fact, by the completion of the study, their average bodyweights exceeded their pre-study scale readout by over 10 percent.

It needs to be emphasized that neither the food obsession of the volunteers nor their refeeding behaviour was the least bit abnormal. To survive, anyone placed in their position, experiencing caloric deprivation as they had, for as long as they volunteered to, would develop an increased sensation of hunger and single-mindedness about eating.[138] Although the volunteers in the Minnesota Starvation Study eventually gained back their lost weight, their body compositions had changed from lean and fit to fat and flabby. Body fat measurements performed after the rapid weight regain phase showed that the participants' lean body mass had substantially decreased throughout the study, while their percentage of body fat had significantly increased.

Death by Yo-Yo

Losing a great deal of weight by some intense dietary means, and then gaining it all back again in short order is hard on the body, let alone on morale and wardrobe choices. Repeated weight loss followed by weight regain is referred to as *weight cycling* and is a common scenario. Canadian National surveys estimate that of the obese adults who have attempted to lose weight, nearly 40 percent of them have a history of weight cycling.[139] Celebrities appear to be particularly prone to this problem. Stars like Jessica Simpson, Janet Jackson, and Matthew Perry have all fallen victim to the feast and famine school of dieting, piling on pounds, then shedding them; and then there's poor Oprah, who seems to be a different size on every cover of the monthly *'O'* Magazine. Such is the cost of stardom. But the problem with weight cycling is more serious than having an unflattering swimsuit photo appear in the *National Enquirer*. Repeated fluctuations in body weight, particularly if extreme, are counterproductive to healthy weight maintenance and can increase the risk of vascular disease.

A Montreal research group demonstrated that weight cycling can lead to changes in body composition—increasing fat stores and decreasing muscle tissue—similar to what was seen in the Minnesota Starvation Study, as well as to a reduction in metabolic rate.[140] They studied two groups of postmenopausal women. The first group had stable weight (the non-weight cyclers), and the second group had a history of significant weight fluctuations, exceeding 10 kg (22 lbs) on at least four separate occasions (the weight cyclers). When they compared the body composition and metabolic rates of members in both groups over time, they found that waist circumference measurements were significantly greater in the weight cyclers and resting metabolic rates significantly lower than in the non-weight cycling group (fig. 6.1). This means that with every repeated loss and regain of weight, it becomes increasingly difficult to maintain a healthy weight. The longer this *yo-yo dieting* goes on, the more fat-burning muscle tissue gets lost, and the slower the calorie-consuming metabolic fire burns. If we want to prevent this downward spiral of muscle loss, we need to go slow and steady with our weight loss measures, ideally losing about half a pound per week and no more than two pounds per week. Anything faster is folly.

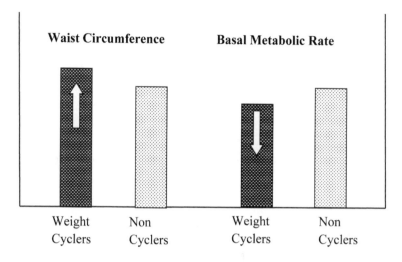

Fig. 6.1 Weight Cycling Worsens Waist Circumference and Metabolic Rate

The problem with weight cycling also goes beyond concerns about achieving ideal body weight. Studies have shown that people who have wide fluctuations in their weight are at a higher risk for serious health troubles, including the development of the metabolic syndrome,[141] diabetes mellitus, and heart disease.[142] In the Iowa Women's Study, those with a history of large weight fluctuations, exceeding 10 percent of their body weight, were at higher risk for premature death.[143] And this isn't just a woman's issue. Epidemiological studies have shown that men who have a history of significant weight cycling are also at increased risk of developing premature vascular disease and dying from heart disease.[144] Both overeating and undereating are potentially dangerous in the long term.

If we want to affect our body weight set point, and permanently lower it, we need to adopt Nietzsche's "long obedience in the same direction" strategy. Being overweight is not merely a caloric issue that's going to be solved by adhering to some restrictive dietary program for a month. This is because the problem with weight gain and obesity isn't merely excess calorie intake, rather it's due to excess insulin levels. Regardless of the diet chosen, to reduce our body weight set point, we need to reduce the fat-promoting hormone, insulin. If we can lower our insulin levels—by avoiding sugar and refined carbs, eating portioned meals, eating less often, exercising regularly, and even fasting intermittently—we can begin to move our body from fat-storage mode, to fat-burning mode. We need to be patient with ourselves. It took time to put on the excess weight; it'll require some time to take it off. How much time is an individual matter, and will depend upon starting your weight and weight loss goals. Resetting our body weight set point is possible, but it requires permanent lifestyle changes, not temporary quick fixes. There's just no avoiding the reality that to achieve sustained weight loss, discipline is essential. Whatever dietary adjustments we make, they need to be adjustments that we can continue to make... forever. So, rather than settling for some short-sighted extreme approach to weight loss like the detox diets offer, we need to adopt a long-range plan with realistic and sustainable weight loss targets focusing on prudent food choices, healthy snacks included.

Will the Real Toxins Please Stand Up!

If we want to identify the bona fide toxins that promote obesity and cardiovascular disease, we need look no further than the processed offerings lining the aisles of our neighbourhood grocery stores. Processed foods are infused with high levels of proven harmful ingredients that can derail weight loss efforts and foster vascular disease.[145] Three notorious processed food ingredients deserve some special mention and our extreme caution.

High Fructose Corn Syrup (HFCS)

In the 1970s, food manufacturers invented a sweetener called high fructose corn syrup, or HFCS for short. When compared to sucrose, HFCS was sweeter, cheaper, more stable and easier to use in food processing.[146] The problem is, however, that HFCS adds empty calories. Often referred to as modified corn syrup on food labels, this man-made marvel is added to a staggering number of foods, increasing the calorie content of innocent-appearing products such as ketchup, pasta sauce, crackers, cereal, commercial white bread, juices, sports drinks, and energy and vitamin water drinks. As a result, it's become increasingly easy to consume a sizeable number of calories and not even know you've done it. The consumption of HFCS has increased by over

1000 percent between 1970 and 1990, far exceeding the changes in intake of any other food or food group.[147] HFCS is the sole caloric sweetener used in soft drinks in the United States, making up over 40 percent of caloric sweeteners added to foods and beverages, and contributing significantly to our culture's sweet tooth and growing waistline. But, the talons of HFCS dig deeper still. This toxic sweetener causes vascular inflammation and insulin resistance, increasing the risk of high blood pressure, type 2 diabetes, and heart artery disease.[148]

Part of the reason for the success of HFCS is that it's an addictive chemical. Animal studies have demonstrated that HFCS can produce addictive behaviour that's as intense as that caused by heroin.[149] Imaging studies in humans have shown that this refined sugar can stimulate the *mesocorticolimbic* portion of the brain referred to as the reward circuit or pleasure pathway.[150] It's the same bit of neurocircuitry that alcohol, nicotine, cocaine and heroin all mess with as they establish their addictive hold on our minds. Eating a sugar-laden snack is analogous to a nicotine addict smoking a cigarette. Both the sugar and the nicotine enter the brain very quickly and stimulate the pleasure pathway, causing the release of the neurotransmitter, dopamine, thereby resulting in a general sense of relief and calm. But, once the sugar or nicotine levels drop off in the blood, our brains are triggered to do the *Oliver Twist* maneuver and ask, "Can I have some more please, sir?" Just as the smoker needs to understand that the cigarette smoked an hour ago is what's causing the present nic-fit, so, too, it's critical to appreciate that our present tummy grumblings and burning desire for something sweet are the direct result of the Kit Kat we ate earlier in the afternoon. Eating fresh fruit and raw vegetables can help break the sugar cycle since they don't activate the pleasure pathway and won't promote food addiction. The natural sugar in fresh produce is absorbed more slowly and, together with the bulkiness of the food, provides a longer sense of satiety. As well, because fruits and vegetables keep company with such an extensive array of essential micronutrients and fiber, our cardiovascular health and weight control efforts are bolstered every time we choose an apple over an apple fritter. Not everything edible is capable of promoting addiction. There are no case reports of broccoli junkies, for example, or apple addicts. When it comes to food addiction, fresh fruit and raw vegetables remain safe territory.

Trans-Fatty Acids

Trans-fat (or hydrogenated fat) is a man-made substance that doesn't exist in nature. Rather, it is vegetable oil infused with hydrogen under high temperatures. It was designed as the answer to the food manufacturers' wish for a clean-burning frying oil that's inexpensive, avoids the use of the blacklisted saturated fats, and has an increased shelf life. And then, there was the unexpected benefit: food manufacturers were able to use trans-fatty acids to expand the number of taste opportunities available to the bored palates of

North Americans, like Oreo cookies and Reeses Peanut Butter Cups. As a result, significant quantities of trans-fat have found their way into a vast number of processed foodstuffs, including cookies, doughnuts, biscuits, chips, nachos, pies, French fries, and movie theatre popcorn. But beware. When it comes to cardiovascular health, trans-fatty acids are the worst thing.151 They destabilize the plaques within the walls of our arteries by increasing the bad LDL cholesterol levels and reducing the good HDL levels, the polar opposite of what we're desperately trying to achieve. Since trans-fatty acids have been identified as accomplices in causing cardiovascular disease, the U.S. Food and Drug Administration now requires that food companies list trans-fats on their nutritional labels. Although this is an important step forward for health awareness, don't believe everything you read; products branded as zero percent (0%) trans-fat are still allowed to contain up to 2.2 grams of this deadly substance.

Sodium or Salt

This innocent-appearing white granular crystal, which sits quietly in shakers on most dining tables across the continent, isn't so innocent. Adding salt to our food adds insult to our blood vessels. Specifically, salt raises blood pressure, which in turn injures the inner lining of our blood vessels. Salt is the single most common cause of high blood pressure in North America, which, in turn, contributes to one-half of all heart attacks and two-thirds of all strokes on the planet.[152] Considering that high blood pressure is the most important factor contributing to heart disease—more important than cigarette smoking—then we can begin to see the enormity of the problem.[153] It's been estimated that if the average salt intake were reduced by half, over 2.5 million stroke and heart attack deaths could be prevented every year worldwide.[154] The concerns with salt may even extend beyond hypertension. Research suggests that salt affects our gut-brain axis and in so doing, produces no end of mayhem—from Parkinson's disease to irritable bowel syndrome.[155] So, new therapeutic targets for countering stroke—the second leading cause of death worldwide—and cognitive dysfunction have been developed. Reducing salt intake applies to people around the globe, as nearly every adult consumes too much salt: on average 9–12 grams per day or around twice the recommended maximum level of intake (5 grams) by the World Health Organization. So, the obvious solution is to avoid salty foods. However, in our salt-laden society, this means doing more than giving up the gherkins. Most of our dietary sodium comes from packaged or processed foods. For example, a single serving of plain pasta may contain only 5 mg of sodium; pretty harmless. But when the food manufacturers get a hold of it, add in their signature "Mamma Mia" tomato sauce, and package it up with a picture of Michelangelo's *David* on the front of the carton, that same serving size of pasta contains Goliath quantities of salt, in some cases over 800 mg of sodium—160 times the original amount!

To stop hypertension, it's not enough to throw out our salt shakers (although, this is an excellent first step); we also need to choose foods that contain less salt. To seriously reduce our salt intake we need to seriously reduce our processed food consumption, particularly the salty varieties. Read the food labels carefully and look for the milligrams of sodium per serving in packaged foods. Anything with over 400 milligrams of sodium per serving needs to be cleared out of your pantry and avoided like the plague (table 6.1). If we want to keep within the daily recommended consumption of 1,200 to 2,300 milligrams of sodium (and, for our cardiovascular health we must try), then even items with sodium content in the 200 to 400 milligrams per serving range should be used sparingly, if at all. Keep this in mind as a general rule when you're filling your grocery cart: if it's packaged and processed, it's too salty, so say "no," put it back on the shelf, and keep walking; but if it's still in Mother Nature's packaging, like unadulterated apples, oranges, carrots, spinach, zucchini, melons, bananas, cherries, or pomegranates… all just waiting there patiently in the produce section, then it's low in salt, so, "yes," go ahead and indulge.

Low Salt (< 200 mg sodium per serving)	High Salt (> 400mg sodium per serving)
Fruits and Vegetables (fresh, dried or frozen)	Pasta Sauces, Canned or Frozen Vegetables in Sauce
Couscous	Packaged Noodle Entrees and Sides
Ricotta Cheese	Most Other Cheeses
Peas, lentils, beans	Canned Pork and Beans, Packaged Rice Side Dishes, Pickles, Anchovies, Olives
Fresh Fish	Canned Smoked Fish
Poultry, fresh meat, eggs	Sausage, Bacon, Canned or Smoked Meats
Seeds, Unsalted Nuts, Hot-air Plain Popcorn	Salted Nuts, Popcorn
Vinegar	Soy Sauce, Condiments

Table 6.1 Low Salt vs. High Salt Food Choices

Offensive Snack Line

Reading package labels can help identify which processed items contain the highest amounts of harmful ingredients, but such scrutiny can be challenging, and not just because of the small print. Packaged food labels can be deceptive! Boldfaced claims like *reduced salt* or *light in sodium* plastered on the packaging simply mean *comparably* less salt, and not by any means, low in salt. Labels like *unsalted* and *no added salt* don't mean salt-free either, but only that no salt was added to the item during processing. Peanuts, canned vegetables, butter, and microwave popcorn are all examples of salty foods labelled in this manner. A label that says *no fat* doesn't mean there isn't a motherlode of sugar inside the package—and *no cholesterol* doesn't mean no fat. And, if the misleading terminology isn't bad enough, then there's the lengthy list of unpronounceable ingredients—enough to tongue-tie a biochemist. Items like propylene glycol alginate or sodium aluminosilicate should probably best be kept on the laboratory shelf, not in our pantry cupboards. Do we really need all those additives, modifiers, emulsifiers, stabilizers, anti-foaming agents, and color fixatives in our food? To meet the bottom line and to sell products capable of sitting on the shelf for eons, maybe, but we certainly don't need such a chemical consommé for health's sake.

Michael Pollan's caution, "Don't eat anything with more than five ingredients on the label" is sage advice.[156] But, when choosing a snack, I would suggest taking his recommendation one step further, and avoid buying anything at all that has a label affixed to it. In other words, don't buy any packaged and processed snack food. Instead, choose snacks that are packaged by Mother Nature with rinds, skins, and peels, over in the produce section. That way, you'll be less likely to confuse processed food with real food. Here's my suggestion: when the afternoon rolls around and you've got a longing for something to fill the void, choose a snack of either fresh fruit or raw vegetables or both, and that's it, nothing else, and no exceptions.

"Oh, come on now! Have you gone completely mad, Doctor, and turned back into Mr. Hyde or something?" you might ask, flabbergasted at my audacious proposal. "Why, there are plenty of snack offerings to choose from besides fruit and vegetables that are still healthy for you. Take low-fat yogurt, for instance, or fat-free cheese, low-sodium sliced turkey breast, whole-grain bread, almonds, and raisins... they're all healthy choices, and the list goes on and on, just ask any self-respecting dietician, and they'll tell you so."

There may indeed be a small handful of healthy snack options that fall beyond the limits of fresh fruit and vegetables. But, here's the thing: we are in a time of crisis—and I'm not referring to climate change or the economic fallout from COVID-19. Diabetes, high blood pressure, heart disease, and stroke are all on the rise, all over the world. As for the obesity statistics (better brace yourself), obesity is associated with more health problems and illness than either smoking, or alcoholism, or poverty, and if current trends continue, obesity may even overtake cigarette smoking as the number one cause of preventable death in North America.[157] Taken together, our society is in such a precarious health position, that we are threatening to undermine all of the cardiovascular health improvements achieved over the past three decades. The possibility has been raised that the rapidly increasing numbers of severely obese children and youth may reverse our modern era's trend of a steady increase in life expectancy. As the direct result of unhealthy lifestyles, our present youth may represent the very first generation in modern history to live shorter lives than their parents.[158] In the understated words of the Apollo 13 astronaut Jim Lovell, "Houston, we've got a problem."

Weight control is an enormous societal problem, but it's not insurmountable, particularly for the motivated individual. The Prussian general Carl von Clausewitzadage got it right when he said, "the best defense is a good offense," and his adage holds true for more than just fighting and football. By intentionally planning a snack into our daily schedule, we can address several important dietary challenges, bearing in mind, of course, that it can't be just any kind of snack. To win the battle of the bulge, we need to attack the snack with well-timed healthy choices that optimize nutrition and minimize calories. The following are four key characteristics that define a healthy snack. For ease of memory, I've fashioned them around the acronym *SAFE* (table 6.2), and encourage my patients to protect themselves from STD's (*Snacking Transmitted Diseases*) by practicing SAFE snacks!

S	Strategically-Timed
A	All-Natural
F	Fiber-Rich
E	Energizing 'Eau'

Table 6.2 Ensuring Safe Snacks

Strategically-Timed

Although there isn't complete uniformity of opinion in the scientific literature regarding optimal meal or snack frequency, the American Dietetic Association recommends four to five small meals/snacks per day including breakfast.[159] And, there's a sound rationale for such an approach: increasing meal frequency with healthy snacking has been shown to help prevent gorging behaviour and improve appetite control.[160] When we eat more frequently, such as every two to three hours, we reduce the power that food has on our thoughts. So, freed from the obsession of eating and thinking about eating, we can turn off the food channel and get on with higher thoughts, like planning a biking route for tomorrow's commute to work. Evenly-spaced healthy snack choices can help maintain our sense of satiety, and reduce the likelihood that we'll make poor dietary choices.-

The Canada Food Guide recommends seven to ten servings of fruit and vegetables every day, where a serving is defined as a medium-sized piece of fruit or half a cup of fresh vegetables. Try eating all ten servings in just one sitting without feeling uncomfortably bloated! The best way we can physically eat low energy, bulky selections is to space them out over the day in the form of strategically planned meals and snacks. Since my work schedule doesn't permit evenly-spaced snacking, I get my fruits and veggie quota during two strategically-timed breaks in my day—one in the mid-morning, and one in the late afternoon. For my mid-morning break, usually an hour or so before lunch, I eat an apple, orange, or banana, or sometimes all three. This has the advantage of not only providing my body with essential nutrients and extra water, but it diminishes my appetite for my lunch meal. The fiber-rich bulky nature of the snack fills my stomach, activating the gastric stretch receptors lining its surface, and produces a level of satiety. Although I don't skip lunch, I find myself eating less and lean, rather than further and fatty. Likewise, I have a single snack in the late afternoon, timed about an hour and a half to two hours before dinnertime. For this pre-dinner snack, I use a 4-cup Tupperware container and fill it with a raw vegetable medley of baby carrots, peas, some cherry tomatoes, and chunks of celery, green pepper, and mini-cucumbers. I don't use any dips or processed adulterations and enjoy the fresh crunch of it all. Similar to my dampened lunch appetite, partaking in a fiber-rich late afternoon snack means that I'm never ravenous for dinner. This spoiling of my appetite, so-called, functions as a natural form of portion control. There's no need for invoking harsh self-restraint. I refrain from overindulging, not because the food isn't tasty, but simply because I'm full. So, when my wife asks who wants seconds, all hands go up but mine. I'm content with a single course and leave the rest for my growing boys to devour.

All-Natural

It's clear. The data is all in and the studies are completed. Despite some persistent passionate Keto-diet debates surrounding the age-old question, "What should I eat, today?" there is one recommendation in the dietary literature that resonates loud and clear: eat your fruits and veggies! What might sound a lot like Mom nagging is actually based on sound evidence—a towering tome of evidence, linking fruit and vegetable consumption to a lengthy list of health benefits, cardiovascular benefits included.[161] While keto-dieters are correct in saying that fruits and vegetables contain carbohydrates, they take things too far when they suggest avoiding these natural offerings just because of the carb content. It's important not to demonize all carbohydrates. In addition to structure—simple vs. complex—the company the carbohydrate keeps can make a significant nutritional difference. Rapidly absorbed simple sugars found in a Twinkie, for example, are not comparable to those in grapefruit or garden carrots. Like the mantra, "location, location, location" used to emphasize the importance of where to invest in real estate, context is key for carbs, as well. The nutrient value of fruits and vegetables more than makeup for the carb count. Cut out potato chips and pretzels, by all means, but don't avoid the benefits of fruits and vegetables just because of the accompanying carbohydrates.

Our cardiovascular system depends upon the nutritional elements found in fruit and vegetables. The inner lining of our blood vessel walls (the endothelium), is under constant attack from the wear and tear of life's pressures: hypertension, elevated LDL cholesterol, and that third piece of pizza you snacked on during your Netflix binge last night. One of the central mechanisms of vascular injury is oxidation. It's the same sort of process that causes your sliced apple to turn brown when left on the counter or your Dodge Durango wheel wells to rust in the winter months. To maintain vascular health, the endothelial cells that line our blood vessels need to counter the oxidation reactions that are normally occurring on their cell surfaces by releasing a powerful anti-oxidant, nitric oxide. Dietary antioxidants including Flavanoids, Carotenoids, and Vitamin C—supplied amply in our friendly neighbourhood fruits and vegetables— can be invaluable in assisting this process. It isn't the only reason to eat fresh produce, but it's one that your heart will continue to beat happily for.

The converse is also true. By favouring food quantity, like that jumbo bag of taco chips on your counter over food quality, like a bowl of blueberries and peaches, we place our cardiovascular system in jeopardy. Even though the majority of North American adults consume more food calories than they can burn in a day (and then some), they often don't consume the right sort of calories and are unable to deliver the much needed antioxidant reinforcements for fighting the blood vessel battle against oxidation. Sadly, just because an excessive amount of energy is being consumed, doesn't mean that micronutrient needs are being met. Despite the incredibly diverse food supply around us, many people fail to reach the bare minimum daily recommendations for fruits and vegetables and, therefore, vitamins and minerals. This unbalanced dietary approach has created a whole new form of undernourishment in our land of plenty called high-calorie malnutrition, with serious cardiovascular and weight control implications.[162]

While we're all at risk for micronutrient deficiencies,

if we eat nutrient-poor selections, the risks are greater for those who are overweight and obese. This is because the amount of fat tissue we have onboard affects the absorption, distribution, metabolism, and excretion of micronutrients, including such critical dietary minerals as iron, zinc, selenium, and magnesium.[163] A British research group noticed that when they applied a nutritional screening tool to a group of hospitalized patients, over 10 percent of the obese patients studied were at high risk for malnutrition.[164] In another study, over 50 percent of morbidly obese patients were found to have vitamin deficiencies during their pre-bariatric surgical assessments.[165] It's ironic, but no less concerning, that the same person could be overweight and undernourished.

One approach to address malnutrition is to reach for dietary supplements and vitamins. While there may be a role for vitamin supplementation in selected cases, particularly during pregnancy and lactation, when nutritional needs are highest, vitamins can't be expected to compensate for ongoing poor dietary choices. As well, overconsumption of various vitamins and supplements may even have detrimental effects on health.[166] Before embarking on a treatment plan, the benefits of taking supplements need to be weighed against the potential risks (including expense) and be reviewed with a family physician. This is especially the case since the evidence for cardiovascular benefit with vitamin therapy is pretty thin. Large epidemiological studies have failed to demonstrate any reduction in heart attack or stroke event rates when vitamin supplementation is rigorously followed.[167] Of course, all that really means is that the health benefits of eating an orange or celery stick exceed those of consuming their vitamin constituents. While food scientists have identified a long list of ingredients in fruits and vegetables, including vitamins, folate, carotenoids, flavenoids, calcium, magnesium, potassium, iron, zinc, and resveratrol, that likely play important roles in health maintenance, it's complete arrogance to think that we know it all or that we can now assemble a miracle pill with all the essentials in it! There's more mystery in a carrot than we'll ever fully understand. Similar to the insight of Shakespeare's *Hamlet*, who said to his friend, "There are more things in heaven and earth, Horatio, than are dreamt of in your philosophy," so, too, our elegant pathophysiological frameworks and molecular approaches to nutrition pale next to the provisions found in the natural world. Eating whole foods, rather than individual nutrients, is always a better approach to building health and controlling weight.

Fiber-Rich

Fresh fruits and raw vegetables are an excellent source of fiber, second only to beans and bran. The health benefits of consuming dietary fiber are well-attested in the scientific literature. They include enhanced functioning of our blood vessels, lowering of bad LDL-cholesterol levels, stabilization of blood sugar and insulin levels, better control of our blood pressure and weight,[168] a reduction in the risk of developing diabetes mellitus and certain cancers, as well as an impressive 20 to 30 percent reduction in the risk of developing heart disease and stroke.[169] The two types of fiber include soluble fiber (also known as dietary or fermentable fiber), found in fruits, vegetables, and legumes; and insoluble fiber, plentiful in whole grains and seeds. Fiber can be thought of as the ingested bits of plants or grains that resist digestion in the upper gastrointestinal tract and, in the words of Jim Morrison, "break on through to the other side." Fiber resists digestion because we lack the enzyme machinery to break it down any further. Herbivores, and even termites, can, but we don't have what it takes to dismantle cellulose, hemicellulose, pectins, and gums. As a result, fiber adds water and bulk to the stool and acts as nature's laxative (second only to public speaking).

Although fiber isn't absorbed across our gastrointestinal lining and into our bloodstream, it does a lot more than prevent us from being *farfrompoopin* (pardon my German). To begin with, fiber doesn't make the transit from one end of our gastrointestinal tract to the other on its lonesome. Fiber interacts with our non-fibrous foods, various breakdown products of digestion, and the bacteria that call our colon home. The components of fiber can bind onto intestinal substances including a variety of undesirables, like bile acids and toxic breakdown products, and take them to the flusher where they belong. Rather than allow potential carcinogens the opportunity to cause injury, fiber binds with them and decreases the amount of time they have in contact with our vulnerable bowels, thereby reducing the risk of colon cancer. As well, since our livers use reabsorbed bile acid as the building block for making cholesterol, fiber's binding of bile leads to a reduction in our serum cholesterol levels. This is good news for our hearts. The lining of our blood vessel walls is exquisitely sensitive to the damaging effects of cholesterol. High fiber diets are important players in the cholesterol-lowering campaign and they may be part of the reason that heart disease and stroke rates are lowered by those who get stuffed with roughage. Although it can be a challenge to get in those recommended seven to nine daily fruit and vegetable servings each day, we will have greater success if we choose to morph every snack break into a fruit and vegetable fiber opportunity.

Energizing 'Eau'

You want an energy boost? Before you have another cup of coffee or grab a *Monster* or *Rockstar* energy drink off the shelf, try putting back a tall glass of water; it's surprisingly refreshing. It's because we oftentimes run on the dry side. Healthy snacks can help. Fresh fruits and raw vegetables contain a significant amount of water. In contrast to desert-dry popcorn or parched Pringles, an orange, for example, contains 80 percent water by weight. The added water in fresh produce energizes and can help suppress our appetites, filling our empty stomachs without filling us with empty calories. This is because the sensation of thirst and that of hunger can easily get confused. We may feel hungry, when in actual fact we are dry. So, when in doubt, drink of a tall glass of water before you snack, and see how you feel. Also, our sense of hunger relates in part to the volume of the contents in our stomachs. When our stomachs are empty, specialized cells within our stomach lining release a hormone called ghrelin, which sends hunger signals to our brains. Ghrelin not only stimulates our appetite but also slows metabolism and thereby fosters energy conservation and weight gain. It's an important component of our bodies' defense against starvation and protects our fat stores from combustion during times of caloric deprivation.[170] However, in our present times of food galore—especially junk food— ghrelin acts more like a gremlin and frustrates weight loss efforts. By contrast, when we eat bulky fresh fruit and raw vegetables, we stimulate the stretch receptors lining our stomach and small intestine, and they in turn cause levels of ghrelin to decrease and our hunger pangs to dissipate. Snacking on fresh produce is particularly advantageous between meals when the desire for a little something to tide us over is strongest. Choosing fresh fruit or raw vegetables gives our hands and mouths something to do and provides enough energy boost and hunger relief to see us through to the next meal.

"How Much Fiber is Enough?"

Well, if you have to ask, then you're probably not eating enough fiber. The usual recommendation is something in the range of 25 to 35 grams of fiber per day, which is substantially more than the 7 grams or less that average North Americans typically consume.[171] Dr. Mehmet Oz, of Oprah fame, addressed the problem of measuring one's daily intake of fiber in some detail when he was describing the health benefits of adopting a high-fiber gorilla diet—the ingestion of eleven pounds of fruits and vegetables per day! Dr. Oz recommended that America should cast a backward glance before flushing and use stool shape to answer the question about fiber adequacy. According to his analysis, if the stool is shaped like an S or C and floats nicely in the bowl, then you've got enough fiber going for you. The curved shape suggests that the stool is loose enough to exit from the colon without the need for labour and delivery. And since fiber binds onto fat and fat is less dense than water, the floating characteristic implies fat content in the stool and successful fat elimination from the body. By contrast, if the stool is straight and narrow, and sinks like a rock to the bottom of the bowl, then more fiber is needed.

This stool assessment technique for determining fiber sufficiency isn't a new one. Dr. Denis Parsons Burkitt, author of the 1979 bestseller, *Don't Forget Fiber in Your Diet,* favoured this approach back in the 1950s. Although complex formulas were already available to help calculate the metabolic equivalents in food and determine optimal dietary fiber intake, Dr. Burkitt didn't have much time for them and believed that stool shape and consistency were a far more accurate test of fiber adequacy. He was a pioneer in the field of dietary fiber and gained his insights, not from mainstream medicine, nor from reading breakfast cereal boxes, but from Sub-Saharan Africa. By examining the diet of African villagers, as well as their feces, Burkitt determined that it was the massive amounts of fiber they consumed that protected them from the scourges of the Western world, including our number one killer, vascular disease. Burt Bacharach's sentimental view of love notwithstanding, Burkitt figured that "what the world needs now is fiber, more fiber." And although he never put his ideas to music, Burkitt felt that the western diet was extremely fiber poor, and spent the remainder of his professional years expounding the benefits of dietary fiber. It is said that during his lecture circuits, Burkitt would drive home his points by showing slides. First, he would project an image of a Westerner's well-formed hard little stool sitting in the bottom of a toilet bowl. Then, for comparison sake, he would show a photo of an African's stool, which resembled more closely a cow pie than anything with a defined shape. So, if you're wondering whether or not you're eating enough fiber, forget the S or C shape, and aim for soft and mushy, instead, and try to bend it like Burkitt!

The sugar-coated processed fiber offerings in our supermarkets, all claiming to provide us with our daily requirements of dietary fiber, are a far cry from the fiber-rich diets Burkitt observed and later recommended. While the food industry has played up the health benefits of fiber, adding a pinch to their processed commodities and claiming they'll reduce the risk of disease with the best of the fiber-fighters, this is more hype than help. It needs to be emphasized that fiber is most beneficial in its unprocessed state. Once broken down, milled, refined, chopped up, boiled, reduced, or pulverized, the fiber that's left behind no longer acts as fiber should. By definition, processed food is fiber poor. If it's packaged, it's probably not a good source of fiber; so, put it back on the shelf and make a beeline to the fresh produce and whole foods section.

Promoting Safe Snacks

"It's true," I agreed with Marion. "Snacking is an established risk factor for developing obesity. However, we shouldn't paint all snacks with the same dismissive brush stroke. By giving some thought to our snack choices and their timing, snacking behaviour can work in our favour, both for abdominal fat reduction and for cardiovascular risk reduction."

"Oh, really, how so?" she asked with interest.

"An afternoon snack of a piece of fruit or some raw vegetables, for example, provides needed nutrients for blood vessel health and dulls hunger grumblings, protecting us from eating junk food during the day or too much food during dinner," I explained.

"I get my vitamins and nutrients by drinking fruit juice and vitamin drinks," she said. "It's easier to pack a bottle of *Glaceau* in my bag than bring fresh produce to work."

"Fruit drinks and so-called vitamin drinks are sources of unwanted sugar calories more than essential vitamins," I countered. "Despite what the advertisements say, drinking our vitamins isn't the healthiest way to consume them. Vitamins in their natural state with built in fiber are what we really need."

"Well, how about fruit leather?" Marion asked. "I buy organic fruit snacks made with 100 percent fruit from organic apples."

"Don't get fooled by the *organic* adjective that food companies bandy about. Made from organic apples or not, fruit leather is merely a disguised sugar snack. And, like all processed products, they're engineered imitations that we should avoid."

"What do you eat, then?" she asked defensively.

"Nature's own," I replied unashamedly. "I cut up an assortment of raw vegetables into a Tupperware container when I'm putting my lunch together the night before. Then, as I wade through my paperwork pile in the afternoon, I pull out my veggies from the fridge and snack in style."

"You eat raw vegetables... all by themselves... no dip?" Marion asked incredulously. "That sounds simply awful."

"Oh, I love the fresh crunch of it all," I countered. "But, although raw vegetables might be a bit of an acquired taste, it's a taste well-worth acquiring, especially if you want to protect your blood vessels from injury, and give yourself a fighting chance at controlling weight."

Chapter Summary
In Defense of Afternoon Snacking

- Unhealthy snack choices can quickly undo exercise and dietary attempts at weight control
- We need to avoid processed snack foods, particularly if they contain High Fructose Corn Syrup (HFCS), trans-fat, or salt
- Detox diets are more hype than help and not based on scientific evidence
- Food deprivation can sometimes work against weight control efforts
- Obesity is not just excess calories; it's excess fat-promoting insulin levels
- Overly-restrictive diets are difficult to sustain and prone to failure
- The best source of vitamins are in their natural form of fruits and vegetables
- The key elements of a healthy snack can be remembered with the SAFE acronym, which stands for strategically-timed, all-natural, fiber-rich, and

energizing 'eau'

- Timing healthy snacks before lunch and dinner provides natural portion control for meals
- Healthy snack choices are low in calories and high in nutrient content
- Fiber promotes health through a litany of mechanisms even though it's not absorbed
- The water in fresh fruit and vegetables provides an energy boost and dampens appetite

Chapter Notes

135. Vanitallie TB. Ancel Keys: a tribute. Nutr Metab (Lond). 2005 Feb 14;2(1):4.

136. Keys A, Brozek J, Henschel A. Mickelsen O, Taylor HL .The biology of human starvation—Vols I & II, Minneapolis, Univeristy of Minnesota Press, 1950.

137. Kalm LM, Semba RD. They starved so that others be better fed: remembering Ancel Keys and the Minnesota experiment. J Nutr. 2005 Jun;135(6):1347-52.

138. Dulloo AG, Jacquet J, Girardier L. Poststarvation hyperphagia and body fat overshooting in humans: a role for feedback signals from lean and fat tissues. Am J Clin Nutr. 1997 Mar;65(3):717-23.

139. Green KL, Cameron J, Polivy K, Cooper L, Liu L, Leiter L and Heatherton T. Weight dissatisfaction and weight loss attempts among Canadian adults: Canadian Heart Health Surveys Research Group. CMAJ 1997;157(suppl 1):S17-S25.

140. Strychar I, Lavoie ME, Messier L, Karelis AD, Doucet E,

Prud'homme D, Fontaine J, Rabasa-Lhoret R Anthropometric, metabolic, psychosocial, and dietary characteristics of overweight/obese postmenopausal women with a history of weight cycling: a MONET (Montreal Ottawa New Emerging Team) study. Journal of the American Dietetic Association 2009;109:4:718-724.

141. Vergnaud AC, Bertrais S, Oppert JM, Maillard-Teyssier L, Galan P, Hercberg S, Czernichow S. Weight fluctuations and risk for metabolic syndrome in an adult cohort. Int J Obes (Lond). 2008 Feb;32(2):315-21.

142. Brownell KD, Rodin J. Medical, metabolic, and psychological effects of weight cycling. Arch Int Med 1994;154:1325-1330.

143. Folsom SA, French SA, Zheng W, Baxter JE, Jeffrey RW. Weight variability and mortality: the Iowa Women's Health Study. Int J Obes Relat Metab Disord. 1996;20(8):704-709.

144. Rzehak P, Meisinger C, Woelke G, Brasche S, Strube G, Heinrich J. Weight change, weight cycling, and mortality in the ERFORT Male Cohort Study. Eur J Epidemiol. 2007;22(10):665-673.

145. Mente A, de Koning L, Shannon HS, Anand SS. A systematic review of the evidence supporting a causal link between dietary factors and coronary heart disease. Arch Intern Med. 2009 Apr 13;169(7):659-69.

146. White JS. Straight talk about high fructose corn syrup: what it is and what it ain't. Am J Clin Nutr. 2008 Dec;88(6):1716S-1721S.

147. Bray GA, Nielsen SJ, Popkin BM. Consumption of high-fructose corn syrup in beverages may play a role in the epidemic of obesity. Am J Clin Nutr. 2004 Apr;79(4):537-43.

148. Hu FB, Malik VS. Sugar-sweetened beverages and risk of obesity and type 2 diabetes: Epidemiologic evidence. Physiol Behav Feb 2010.

149. Avena NM. Examining the addictive-like properties of binge eating using an animal model of sugar dependence. Exp Clin Psychopharmacol. 2007 Oct;15(5):481-91.

150. Wang GJ, Volkow ND, Thanos PK, Fowler JS. Similarity between obesity and drug addiction as assessed by neurofunctional imaging: a concept review. J Addict Dis. 2004;23(3):39-53.

151. Mozaffarian D, Katan ME, Ascherio A, Stampfer MJ, Willett WC. Trans fatty acids and cardiovascular disease. N Engl J Med 2006;354: 1601-13.

152. Whitworth JA. 2003 World Health Organization (WHO/International Society of Hypertension (ISH) statement on management of hypertension. J Hypertens 2003;21:1983-92.

153. World Health Organization. International Coronary Heart Disease Mortality Trends in Men, 1968-2003;Statistics;2005.

154. Padwal, RS, Hemmelgarn BR, Khan NA, et al: for the Canadian Hypertension Education Program. The 2009 CHEP recommendations for the management of hypertension: Part 1—blood pressure measurement, diagnosis, and assessment of risk. J Cardiol 2009;25(5):279-286.

155. Faraco, G et al. Nat Neurosci. 2018 Feb; 21(2): 240–249.

156. Michael Pollan. In Defense of Food: An Eater's Manifesto. Penguin Press 2008.

157. Sturm R, Well KB. Does obesity contribute as much to morbidity as poverty or smoking? Public Health 2001;115:229-35.

158. Daniels SR. The consequences of childhood overweight and obesity. Future Child. 2006 Spring;16(1):47-67.

159. Seagle HM, Strain GW, Makris A, Reeves RS; American Dietetic Association. Position of the American Dietetic Association: weight management. J Am Diet Assoc. 2009

Feb;109(2):330-46.

160. Speechly DP, Bufferstein R. Greater appetite control associated with an increased frequency of eating in lean males. Appetite 1999;33:285-297.

161. Ignarro LJ, Balestrieri ML, Napoli C. Nutrition, physical activity, and cardiovascular disease: an update. Cardiovasc Res. 2007 Jan 15;73(2):326-40.

162. Kaidar-Person O, Person B, Szomstein S, Rosenthal RJ. Nutritional deficiencies in morbidly obese patients: a new form of malnutrition? Part A: vitamins. Obes Surg. 2008 Jul;18(7):870-6.

163. Gibson RS. The role of diet and host-related factors in nutrient bioavailability and thus in nutrient-based dietary requirement estimates. Food Nutr Bull. 2007 Mar;28(1 Suppl International):S77-100.

164. Lamb CA, Parr J, Lamb EI, Warren MD. Adult malnutrition screening, prevalence and management in a United Kingdom hospital: cross-sectional study. Br J Nutr. 2009 Feb 10:1-5.

165. Toh SY, Zarshenas N, Jorgensen J. Prevalence of nutrient deficiencies in bariatric patients. Nutrition. 2009 May 30.

166. Labbe RF. Dangers of iron and vitamin C supplements. J Am Diet Assoc. 1993 May;93(5):526-7.

167. Marchioli R, Schweiger C, Levantesi G, Tavazzi L, Valagussa F. Antioxidant vitamins and prevention of cardiovascular disease: epidemiological and clinical trial data. Lipids. 2001;36 Suppl:S53-63.

168. Khan NA, Hemmelgarn B, Herman RJ, Bell CM,et al. The 2009 Canadian Hypertension Education Program recommendations for the management of hypertension: Part 2--therapy. Can J Cardiol. 2009 May;25(5):287-98.

169. Salas-Salvadó J, Bulló M, Pérez-Heras A, Ros E. Dietary

fiber, nuts and cardiovascular diseases. Br J Nutr. 2006 Nov;96 Suppl 2:S46-51.

170. Wells T. Ghrelin - Defender of fat. Prog Lipid Res. 2009 May 3.

171. Food and Nutrition Board, Institute of Medicine. Dietary reference intakes for energy, carbohydrate, fiber, fat, fatty acids, cholesterol, protein, and amino acids. Washington, DC: National Academy Press; 2002.

Chapter 7
Redefining Fine Dining
Importance of the Family Meal

Every Man for Himself

After scanning over my patient notes to refresh my memory, I entered the patient consultation room and saw Marion standing by the sink, looking at the heart poster on the wall. "Hi there; how are you doing today?" I asked.

"Oh, just fine," she replied, walking over to her chair to take a seat.

"How was your appointment with the dietician?" I asked further.

"Lots of information!" Marion exclaimed. "And she was a lovely person to talk with and easy to understand. She gave me a better sense of how to steer away from all those hidden fats and sugars in the supermarket. Thanks for setting that up for me," she said sincerely.

"I'm glad you found that useful. Dieticians are a wealth of practical information on healthy eating," I said. "So what are you planning for dinner tonight?" I asked, as I fit the blood pressure cuff around her arm.

"I haven't thought that far ahead," Marion laughed.

"And I'm ashamed to say that I haven't cooked a good, old-fashioned dinner in an awfully long time. Last Thanksgiving, probably, and my sister prepared most of that meal," she admitted. "The three meals that I typically serve are frozen, microwave or take out."

"Not much good in knowing about healthy nutrition, if you don't give yourself an opportunity to prepare meals," I smiled. "What do you typically do for dinner then?" I inquired.

"Oh, this and that. I usually leave a few things out for the kids to graze on after school. Since our schedules are so different from each other, individualized meals make more sense. And thank God for the microwave!" Marion exclaimed.

"You mean, you don't eat as a family?" I asked, shuddering at the idea of my own boys helping themselves to whatever, and to the mess they'd predictably leave behind.

"No, with the busy lives we lead, that's just not practical," she said, shaking her head. "Our granddaughters have their midweek volleyball and basketball practices, and dance lessons on Thursdays. And with my daughter's long work hours and my own commute home... well, it's nearly impossible for us to sit down together for a meal," Marion explained with a frown.

"Too bad," I said. "That's my favourite time of the day. It's around the dinner table that I catch up with my boys and connect. Without the dinner ritual, we'd soon be ships passing in the night," I admitted. "How about you and your husband; you must eat together, at least?" I asked.

"Well, Bill loves to watch the news on television, which I find too depressing. So, he usually takes his meal into the living room, while I eat in the kitchen and watch *This is Us*," she said.

"Hmmm... well, the only thing I can imagine that's worse than having a television set turned on during the dinner hour, is having two TVs on," I said, making a facial grimace for emphasis.

"Well, I like to have *some* company when I'm eating dinner," Marion said in defense.

"When it comes to eating, television is bad company. Screen time not only encourages sedentary behavior, it's fattening," I said.

"Fattening? Oh, come on," Marion argued. "I don't see how watching a little TV can affect my weight."

"It's true," I continued. "By exposing us to consumerism and distracting us from food enjoyment, watching television or eating in front of the computer fosters mindless eating and promotes overeating. Studies have demonstrated a direct relationship between screen time and the risk of obesity.[172] So, rather than having your meal with Netflix or your newsfeed, put on some music instead. Use the dinner meal as an opportunity to catch up with your husband. Conversation is the best accompaniment to any meal."

Dinner Unplugged

Media consumption is a distracting enterprise. Mom used to bemoan our television watching, trying in vain to get us children to listen to her while *Starsky and Hutch* were in the middle of a car chase, or when the *Six Million Dollar Man* was finally using his bionic arm. It's even more of an issue today with the steady stream of high-speed internet images bombarding our brains, and creating a veritable hypnotic spell. Media not only captures our imaginations but holds them ransom, while it robs us of our ability to have original thoughts. Studies have shown that screen time can change our brain wave patterns from the alert and orientated "beta" wave type to the more docile and receptive "alpha" waves. It's not the program content so much as the radiant light emitted from the computer screen or boob tube that induces the slower, meditative brain waves on electroencephalogram recordings.[173] It's also been shown that our brain's neurochemistry can be altered by television and the internet, as well. The neurotransmitter, dopamine, gets released into our brain's nerve endings, and the pleasure pathway—that little bit of neuro-circuitry that keeps gamblers gambling, drinkers drinking, smokers smoking, and snorters snorting— gets activated by screen time.[174] In short, high-speed internet and television can be addictive. So, we need to be careful. If media is to have a continued time and place in our lives, then the amount of time and the viewing places need to be well-defined and limited, particularly in relation to mealtimes.

Research has shown that people who frequently eat in front of the screen—be it television or the computer—consistently make two dietary errors: first, they fail to keep to the recommended portion sizes, but prefer larger servings and, second, they opt for unhealthy items like French fries and potato chips rather than making healthy choices like carrot sticks and celery.[175] When all eyes are glued on *Breaking Bad*, it's bad food choices high in fat, salt, and sugar that win out, while fruits and vegetables get kicked off the island.[176] Part of the problem is the distraction of rapid-fire images, but it's even more sinister than this. Advertising, commercials, infomercials, and product placements affect the way we think about food, in general, and about energy-dense, processed food, in particular.[177] Food advertising encourages viewers to eat more than they should and choose the wrong items, which, not surprisingly, promotes obesity. One study suggested that if unhealthy food wasn't advertised on television (and unhealthy food is pretty much the only type of food ever advertised in media), nearly one in three obese children in the United States may not have developed their weight problem.[178] So, if we want to teach our children about healthy eating choices and appropriate portion sizes (while modeling it ourselves while we're at it), then we'll have to power down the computer and keep the TV remote out of hand, especially over the dinner hour.

The Cost of Convenience

Frozen food advocates claim that portion-controlled, commercial meals can be used to re-train people about healthy serving sizes and help prevent overeating. Subscribers to weight loss programs, such as *Jenny Craig*, probably owe much of their success to the limited serving sizes promoted in their meals. However, when the lights are dimmed, the television gets flicked on, and everyone settles into their comfy recliners, serving size boundaries promptly blur, and suddenly, no matter what's being munched on, more is better. We may be able to keep to Miss Piggy's advice to "Never eat more than you can lift," but not much more.

Commercial dinners may be a convenient solution to the "What should I make for supper?" conundrum, but they're no replacement for the good, old fashioned, home-cooked meal Mom used to make us, bless her heart. This is because those dinners are not made with the same care and attention to nutrition that she used. Sappy commercials soaked in sentimentality might have us believe otherwise, harkening us back to simpler times. But in reality, nutrition is not the primary focus of food producers; sales are. Advertisers only give us those sentimental lines because they're concerned with their bottom line. The frozen food industry is a highly competitive business, with hundreds of companies vying for the consumer kitty. To keep in the game, manufacturers need to make their products immediately appealing to a broad range of consumers. They do this by repeatedly adding salt, fat and sugar to their products, because, hey, everyone knows that "lip-smacking" trumps "heart-healthy." So, before you go out and slip a half dozen frozen dinners into your grocery cart, read the package ingredients; you'll be amazed. TV dinners typically contain between 700 and 1,800 milligrams (mg) of sodium per single serving. That amounts to over half of the recommended salt intake for an entire day, which is 2,300 mg (100 mmol of sodium or one teaspoon of table salt).[179]

When it comes to fat content, TV dinners tend to perform as dismally. Regardless of the brand—Stouffer's, Swanson, or Marie Callender's—the amount of fat in a frozen dinner rivals any Big Mac, and that's a big problem. Saturated fat consumption causes direct injury to our blood vessels as it makes its way to our thighs, jowls and waistlines. Accordingly, both the American Heart Association and the Canadian Cardiovascular Society recommend that no more than 7 percent of our calories should derive from saturated fat, less than 1 percent from trans-fat (the absolutely worst kind of fat) and that we keep our daily cholesterol intake to less than 300 milligrams,[180] which is a tall order if all we eat are TV dinners. Even the dinners that are targeted at those with health concerns, including obesity and heart disease, seldom come anywhere close to the bull's eye of health. Food manufacturers tend to provide only a small fraction of the vegetables, fruits, and grains that we need, and make up the difference by generously ladling on the saturated fats, which we don't need. Adding fat calories is a cheap way to satisfy customers, but it's an unhealthy way to eat. Supplementing a frozen-dinner meal with some fresh cut veggies doesn't get around the overconsumption of fat, which is both hard on our blood vessels and our waistlines.

Hamburger Helpless

In the world of packaged and processed, the sky is the limit when it comes to food choices. Whatever type of eating experience we may desire, there's a convenience foodstuff out there just waiting to bring pleasure to our tastebuds. If you don't have a convenience store nearby, don't worry; big fat plans are underway to have fast food outlets open within ten minutes of every citizen on the continent. In our pressure cooker lives, where every moment is measured out with coffee spoons, and where we are under incessant strain to save time, there are certain advantages to eating convenience foods. For starters, they require little or no effort (let alone culinary skill) to prepare, and their use can speed up meal preparation, or, depending on the product, allow us to avoid it altogether. Second, having a choice of separate entrees makes everyone in the family happy; parents can avoid the frustrating battle of getting their kids to "finish what's on your plate, or there's no dessert!" As well, since the production, storage, and sale of industrially prepared food products are subject to strict regulations and controls, properly stored ready-to-use packaged goods are less likely to be sources of bacteria than are fresh goods.

Fast food has never been faster, cheaper or easier. But, if "we are what we eat," then fast, cheap, and easy shouldn't be our primary goals. We've become a take-out, drive-through, on-the-go, dine-alone culture. Convenience food has devalued eating and robbed us of our appreciation for the shared meal. We've made the business of eating so simple that it's become hard to rationalize why we should sit down for a meal as a family. But just because we *can* microwave a meal in two minutes and have it finished in three, doesn't mean we *should* be eating our dinners in this manner. In the cult classic Sci-Fi film, *Silent Running,* we are given a glimpse of the ultimate fast food. Bruce Dern masterfully plays the role of a desperate astronaut caught alone in a battle to save the last of earth's vegetation. Instead of sitting down to a meal of fresh produce like Dern's character continues to encourage, the other astronauts take a few seconds to simply swallow a handful of pills that contain "everything you need." The rich and robust experience of the shared meal is reduced to a meagre skeleton of chemicals and calories. When it comes to food, fast certainly doesn't mean healthy, not for our hearts, and not for our souls.

While convenience foods may be quite useful, especially for the elderly, sick, or handicapped persons, they have, at the same time, reduced the rich heritage of the family meal to little more than a fast food, gotta-run experience. So, before we ditch our recipe books and sell our saucepans, it may be beneficial to consider the cost. And by cost, I'm not merely referring to the obvious expense of buying packaged and processed items (although this can significantly add up). There is also the hidden cost of allowing our tastebuds to be increasingly shaped by the food industry, leading us into a rather unfortunate negative spiral: the more we use convenience foods, the more dependent we become on them, and the more we *need* to use them. Perhaps the most significant cost of our reliance on convenience foods is the erosion of our knowledge of how to select and prepare healthy meals. When it comes to a home-cooked meal, most of us are nearly clueless about where to begin. "How do I boil water again, Honey?.. Okay, okay, okay... and which one is the kettle again?" We've been stocking our pantry with *Campbell's* for so long, we can't remember how to make a soup stock from scratch, even if our lives depended on it (and they just might). Cooking from scratch has moved into a different realm. It's now seen as entertainment, a hobby, or, perhaps, an impractical fancy, all things that most of us don't have time for. This is a sorry state of affairs. Much of who we are as a people is contained in the pages of our shared recipes. With the loss of the home-cooked meal, we begin to lose our cultural traditions, regional customs, and familial heritage and, sadly, we are positioned to leave an impoverished legacy for the generations to come. We are more than what we eat. Let's not trade in our traditions for ten minutes saved here and fewer dishes to wash there.

Dinner Dismantled

The time-honoured tradition of the family meal is an endangered species that is fast approaching extinction. And, while screen time and convenience food dinners may be contributing to the dinner dismantling process, they are by no means the only explanations for dinner's sickly state. Let's consider three additional culprits.

Busy Parents

Less than a third of Canadian children eat with both parents on any given night of the week.[181] Why is this the case? Because both parents are seldom around. While the high divorce rate may be contributing to this sad statistic, it's also in part because 80 percent of married couples in North America are dual income earners. This is the highest rate of double income ever seen in our history and has rendered the dual-income family our current societal norm. When both husband and wife work outside the home in an attempt to provide a consistent income for their families, there are fewer available feet to walk to the market and fewer available hands to prepare the meals. This is an unfortunate reality for many people, making it all the more critical that we don't reduce our time to some commodity that can be bought or sold. One of the hidden blessings of the COVID-19 pandemic with the early *stay-at-home* recommendations, was the mandate for many to work from home. This provided the opportunities for families to once again gather around the dinner table and experience together the richness of the shared meal. Although most of us will need to return to our places of work in some fashion, let's not return to our prior impoverished habits of undervaluing the meal-time. Despite what the business-minded might think, time is worth far more than money. Intentional planning is needed to help prevent our precious family moments—dinnertime moments included—from being snatched away by overly zealous to-do lists and work priorities.

Busy Children

Whatever happened to those days when kids had free time, without a dizzying program of scheduled activities after they came home from school? Gone are the long lazy afternoons of neighborhood fun playing tag, hide-and-seek, "kick the can," "Mother May I," and "Green Light Red Light." In more recent times, children have become so over-committed with after school activities that their parents have come to the verge of being committed. If it's not Conservatory piano lessons or Suzuki violin lessons, then it's karate class, Irish dancing, club soccer, volleyball, or hockey. Rather than having the opportunity to set the dinner table and help prepare the family meal, kids have been scooped up and run across town for their recitals or sport practice times. And as always, the dinner meal takes the hit. In our newly altered COVID world, children's extracurricular activities may be on hold, but they remain busier than ever: not on the playground, but online. They may not be dispersed to every sort of program, but are still dispersed, now on every sort of screen and device. Exceptional are families who make the evening meal a priority and sit down at the dinner table together. More commonly, it's every man for himself, each person eating their individually packaged portion, one finishing while another's starting, resembling more closely a WWF tag-team wrestling match, than a family gathering.

Busy Cities

Cities are growing up and out, and suburbs are growing farther from them, gobbling up precious green space in their path. As a result, commuting times are increasing from short minutes a day to tedious hours. The average urban Canadian spends upwards of one hour commuting to and from work, and this doesn't even include the time spent trying to find parking. That amounts to nearly twelve full days a year wasted travelling between work and home.[182] We would do well to rethink our use of time and consider the difference between the value of *things* and the things of *value*. Long commutes spread us out too thinly for health's sake.

There are formidable obstacles that separate us from gathering at our dinner tables, true enough. But before we surrender to the pressures of this age and exchange our dinner bell for *Taco Bell*, we need to be aware of what's at stake. The consequences of dismantling dinner are serious and far reaching, and will not only negatively affect us, but will misshape and harm generations to come. When children no longer put their feet under the same dinner table as their parents, psychosocial ills come out of the woodwork, potentially including behavioural problems, poor school performance, eating disorders, promiscuity, and drug abuse.[183] It may seem too simple to be true, but the family dinner meal can help protect children from these serious problems, as well as help them develop healthy eating patterns. Studies confirm that regular family meals during the early adolescence years can contribute to the formation of healthy eating habits in adulthood and help curb the exponentially growing obesity crisis.[184] Therefore, we mustn't allow the microwave mindset of this instant gratification culture in which we live to reduce our precious family times to self-serving jiffy moments.

One Diet Fits All?

The dietary landscape in our society seems to be divided paradoxically. On one side, we have the pro-diet territory, where diet reigns supreme, and diet enthusiasts tend to overemphasize the importance of diet on health, often with unproven claims. On the other side, we have the diet-indifferent terrain, where the diet-disillusioned or diet-ignorant folk lean towards undervaluing the role that diet plays on their health. As is so often the case, the truth of the matter lies somewhere in the rocks and crags of the middle ground. Part of the difficulty in negotiating through this middle ground of healthy eating is our misunderstanding of how diet is defined. The enjoyment and simplicity of selecting nutritious foods to sustain life, of body and soul, has been lost in the abyss of our dieting culture. People are initially attracted by the shallow claims of the diet gurus, only to be disappointed after "failing" on yet another dietary regimen. Despite following the diet's strict rules and regulations, they remain bound to their unwanted pounds. For a large number of frustrated dieters, the term DIET has become a four-letter word, conjuring up feelings of guilt and shame. As a result, they may associate the letter *D* in diet with *D*raconian, the *I* with *I*nflexible, the *E* with *E*xpensive, and the *T* with *T*edious. And they have a point; popular diets can be all of these things, and in some cases, can do more harm than good.

To illustrate the inflexibility of fad diets, consider the Greek story of Procrustes. He was a kindly-appearing old man with angel eyes and a long, grey, fatherly beard. His home was positioned along the well-travelled road into Athens, providing him with the opportunity to greet travelers, while sitting on his porch, and smoking his pipe. "Welcome to Athens," he would say to them with his warm and disarming smile. "Come in and rest your weary feet a while." Procrustes appeared to have the gift of hospitality, and many an exhausted visitor took him up on his kind offer. He would feed his travelers barley cakes and figs and pass around wine and cheese after they were finished. "You mustn't leave just yet," he would admonish them. "Relax and stay the night." After all, he had this bed that, he claimed, "would fit everyone... one size fits all... you must see it!" However, what the travelers didn't realize (until it was too late, of course), was just how the fitting and sizing was done. The length of the bed didn't change any, but the visitors' length did. If his guests were tall, with feet dangling out over the end of the bed, Procrustes would take the liberty of cutting pieces off so the length of his visitors would exactly match the length of his bed. And if his guests were short, Procrustes would painstakingly stretch them until their frame equaled the frame of the bed. In the end, everyone was conformed to fit the bed. One size, indeed, fit all.

Too often, the dietary advice that gets propagated is Procrustean. We are told to eat this exact number of calories, according to that magic macronutrient composition, partaking of only these "power foods" and those commercial products, and always at this specific time of day. This sort of inflexible, draconian approach to eating may trim away a few pounds in the short term, but it leaves the dieter, like Procrustes left his visitors, limping and hobbling, and hardly any happier or healthier. How on earth can one diet fit all? Our diverse metabolic needs, ethnic backgrounds, and taste experiences won't allow for it. And there are just too many wonderful food experiences out there to limit ourselves to one dreary regimen. Better is to consider that the *D* in diet stands for Diversity, the *I* with Inexpensive, the *E* with Essential, and the *T* with Timely. Robert Browning said, "A person's reach should exceed their grasp, otherwise what's a heaven for?" Counting calories is fine for a day or two, but restraint only works for so long. We need to find pleasure in life, eating meals included. Otherwise, what's the point of living in a paradise of abundant, healthy food choices, if we can't reach for a taste? Rather than being conformed to a dietary regimen of *shoulds* and *shouldn'ts*, we need to transform diets— ideally, the healthy, proven effective ones—to our tastes, budgets and timetables. It's far healthier to garner guidance from various diets, incorporating their valuable lessons (like "hold the sour cream" and "no Hollandaise sauce for me, thanks") than to reduce our dietary options to some narrow list of edibles. For a reliable source for dietary information, check out the Canada Food Guide (www.hc-sc.gc.ca/fn-an/ food-guide-aliment/index-eng.php), and give some thought to how those recommendations can fit into your meal plans.

A Fistful of Diets

The dismantling of dinner, with the fading away of our family recipes and the erosion of our culinary skills, has made us susceptible to the allure of the diet craze. Without keeping alive our dietary heritage, we become prone to considering other types of diets—perhaps even diets that promise instant weight loss, enhanced sex appeal, or a better job. But choosing which diet to follow to achieve efficient and healthy weight loss, as well as cardiovascular health, is no easy task. To begin with, there are just so many options, and what's more, the gap between scientific evidence and popular opinion is a vast and growing chasm. So, before delving into what reliable dietary evidence does exists, it's important to understand that in the world of dieting, there are not only many means of dieting, but many motivations for doing so. Just as no one diet fits everyone's palate or needs, so too, no one dietary goal inspires every nutritional ambition or eating plan. Although weight loss and dieting are often considered synonymous, this is not always the case. Many diets aren't intended for weight loss at all, and some even have the opposite aim. In underweight elderly patients, for example, a diet that supplements calorie-rich snacks and drinks between meals is employed to stave off advancing frailty. Here, the intent is to increase some meat on the ribs, not decrease. Similarly, bodybuilders consume high-calorie diets during the bulk phase of their training. Their goal is also to gain and not lose. With strict dietary regimens of numerous chicken breasts, copious quantities of eggs, and plenty of protein powders, they aim to meet energy demands in the gym to optimize muscle building. Then, during their 'cut' phase, when body sculpting rather than bulking becomes the goal, they will often follow an extremely low-carb diet, like the Keto Diet, interposed with some intermittent fasting. This macronutrient restriction and calorie shift facilitates the removal of unwanted fat and allows their abdominal six-packs to stand out better, all rippling and ready to grate cheese.

Some diets weren't intended for weight loss at all. Take the gluten-free diet for example. Although popularized in our present-day culture as a weight-reducing method, the gluten-free diet is medicinal by design. Those who benefit the most from avoiding gluten aren't the overweight looking to shed some pounds, but first and foremost, those who suffer from Celiac disease. While some weight loss can occur by cutting out gluten, for Celiac patients, the diet is less about weight control and more about a remedy for their symptoms of gluten-induced intestinal injury.

By comparison, some diets are less about weight and nutrition, and more ideological. The vegan diet, for example, is often adhered to by those motivated less by weight control and more by environmental concerns. Hoping to reduce their carbon footprint, many vegans abstain from meat and dairy products to model a more sustainable dietary approach for the good of the planet. Although there are numerous health benefits from eating vegetarian fare (as well as some risks, such as developing iron deficiency anemia), advocates more commonly promote their restrictive lifestyle as a woke badge of honor, rather than a superior nutritional approach. So, before embarking on a dietary plan (especially an extreme one that may prove challenging to stick with), it's important to ensure that our dietary goals align with the primary purpose of the dietary regimen.

In terms of weight loss, many diets are vying for our attention—gluten-free, Ketogenic, The Paleo Diet, Alkaline Diet, Whole 30, Wheat Belly, The Cleanse, Carb Cycling, The

Subway Diet, The Cabbage Soup Diet.... Where to begin? The vast array of options betray the reality that perhaps there is no best diet to lose weight. To clarify the issue, studies have been done comparing popular weight-reducing diets. One such study included a carbohydrate-restricted diet, a fat-restricted diet, a calorie-restricted diet, and a fat/protein/carbohydrate-balanced diet.[185] Although dietary adherence rates were on the low side, over the one-year study period each of the diets resulted in a modest, but significant, reduction in both weight (roughly between 5 to 7 kg, or 10 to 15 lbs) and LDL-cholesterol levels (around a 10 percent drop). So, in an attempt to tease out which diet might still be superior, the researchers went back to their drawing boards. They compared the macronutrient proportions of each of the main diets (that is, the amount of protein, carbohydrate, and fat in each diet). The researchers ensured that calorie consumption was the same for dieters, regardless of which diet they were assigned to follow. They systematically compared the diets: high fat against low fat; high protein against average protein; high carbohydrate against low carbohydrate. [186] While it's easy to *say* that one diet is best, it's quite another thing to *prove* it so. Despite excellent study design and careful follow-up, not one diet demonstrated superiority. No matter which diet was followed, the weight loss results were remarkably similar. High-fat or low, high-carb or low, no one dietary regimen fared better than another. What was even more disheartening for the competing diets was this: even though the participants paid close attention to the stringent dietary specifications, most, regardless of the diet they followed, remained overweight. Those who lost weight did so by only a modest amount, and "certainly not worth all the effort," many felt.

When the dust settled and the researchers picked through the rubble looking for any surviving nuggets of wisdom from their studies, they came to this conclusion: more important than the diets' proportion of fat, protein or carbohydrate, was the education, support, and encouragement offered to the dieters. It was felt that the counselling during the diet, rather than the composition of the diet, was the more important factor for weight loss success. In this world of attractive, labour-saving devices available at our fingertips and mouth-watering calorie-dense foods within easy reach, maintaining weight, let alone trying to lose weight, isn't easy. While we diet, regardless of what dietary regimen we choose, we need all the support we can get. Even the Lone Ranger had Tonto. So, don't go it alone: always diet in good company.

If You Must Dash, then DASH Diet

For those prone to high blood pressure, The DASH diet (which stands for *The Dietary Approach to Stop Hypertension*) is important to be aware of. High blood pressure affects a third of the Canadian population and, since it's such a major player in the development of cardiovascular disease, we need to do our best to stop hypertension.[187] Our day-to-day dietary choices can help.[188] The landmark study which demonstrated this involved 459 hypertensive adults divided into two groups. One group followed the DASH diet, a diet rich in fruits and vegetables, and items with reduced saturated fat. The second group was allowed to carry on with eating typical North American fare. The participants' blood pressures, which were measured throughout the study, changed significantly. After only two months, the folks on the DASH diet had a considerable drop in blood pressure, while their counterparts experienced the opposite effect. Details about the diet are on the web (www.nhlbi.nih.gov/health/hbp/dash/new-dash.pdf), and to give you an idea of what the diet might look like, a sample dinner menu is listed below (table 7.1).

Food Item	Quantity	Serving Size
herbed baked cod	3 oz	1 fish
scallion rice	1 cup	2 grains
steamed broccoli	1/2 cup	1 vegetable
stewed tomatoes	1/2 cup	1 vegetable
spinach salad: raw spinach cherry tomatoes cucumber	 1/2 cup 2 2 slices	 1 vegetable
light Italian salad dressing	1 Tbsp	1/2 fat
whole wheat dinner roll	1 small	1 grain
soft margarine	1 tsp	1 fat
melon balls	1/2 cup	1 fruit

Table 7.1 Sample DASH Dinner Menu (based on a 2000 calorie daily diet)

Cut to the Core

In terms of coronary artery disease, one diet that deserves to be underscored is Dr. Dean Ornish's fat-restricted diet. Although his diet wasn't shown to be superior to the other popular diets with regard to weight loss, the health benefits of Dr. Ornish's dietary approach transcend weight reduction. He proved in his Lifestyle Heart Trial that eating a high-fiber, low-fat, vegetarian diet not only helps in healthy weight loss efforts, but it can also slow down the progression of vascular plaque buildup on the inside of our arteries.[189] Furthermore, Dr. Ornish demonstrated that his fat-restricted diet actually helps shrink vascular plaques—kind of like what Preparation H does to hemorrhoids, but on our injured blood vessels, instead, and without the need of hourly application. Although following a diet with no meat and with less than 10 percent fat may be a little harder to swallow than the Mediterranean or DASH diets, significant plaque reversal was demonstrated within one year of starting the diet, and plaques were shown to remain stable even after five years.

One of the mechanisms undergirding the phenomenon of plaque buildup and regression involves a little fat molecule called LDL cholesterol, or low-density lipoprotein cholesterol. LDL cholesterol is bad news. It weasels its way through the endothelium and deep into the walls of our blood vessels, getting deposited within the cholesterol core of our vascular plaques (fig. 7.1). The more LDL cholesterol particles we have floating around in our circulation, the greater the size and number of our vascular plaques, and the greater the risk of developing heart artery disease and stroke. The data is overwhelmingly clear: LDL cholesterol is to people as Raid is to bugs; it kills humans dead, and does so in a predictable, dose-dependent fashion, with very few exceptions.

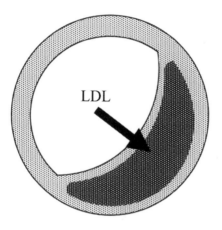

Fig. 7.1 LDL Cholesterol Adds to the Plaque Core

"Well, why can't our bodies do something to stop this process? After all, our immune system fights off viruses. Why can't it fight off LDL cholesterol, too?" some might wonder. To which our weary body puts down its broom and dustpan and answers indignantly, "All day long I scour your blood vessels trying to keep you disease-free, dusting, cleaning, vacuuming, and this is the thanks I get? I'm doing my level best to stop LDL cholesterol from building up in your blood vessels! But you insist on eating all those Nachos and watching all those NHL games. Enough already! I've had it with all your complaining. If avoiding atherosclerosis is so darn important to you, then why don't you do something to help out? And get your feet off the coffee table; I've just polished it!"

Every moment of every day, our dutiful white blood cells cruise the miles upon miles of blood vessels that make up our circulatory system, in a tireless effort to serve our bodies and protect us from disease. Part of their mission is to target areas of vascular plaque and force vascular injury to cease and desist. When they spot trouble, they cordon off the area and commandeer more inflammatory cells to contain the damage. In preparing to enter into the injured zone, they transform themselves into specialized cells called macrophages (or "big eaters"). Armoured with this SWAT gear, they can more readily squeeze into tight places and resist attack. When they come across delinquent LDL cholesterol molecules hanging around, spray painting "heart attacks rule!" or "infarct yourself!" graffiti on our vascular walls, they throw them into their paddy wagon, to haul them downtown for further questioning. But, here's the rub: white blood cells can ingest LDL cholesterol easily enough, but they are unable to render this bad cholesterol harmless. They have no means of breaking down the fat molecule. Our bodies lack the basic machinery to detoxify LDL cholesterol. We can refashion some LDL cholesterol into hormones or excrete it into our bile, but we can't break it down. As a result, the ingested bad fat builds up within the macrophages and poisons them. And the really unfortunate part is this: our white blood cells are unaware of their inability to impair or remove the LDL enemy. So, they just ingest away until it's too late, and then they die, adding to the debris within the cholesterol core of our blood vessel walls.

By contrast to eating foods high in saturated fat, like red meat, TV dinners, and desserts (which increase LDL cholesterol levels and vascular plaque size), following a diet like Dr. Ornish recommends reduces LDL cholesterol levels and brings vascular plaques under control. You don't have to be a vegetarian to enjoy heart health, but it wouldn't hurt. I see very few vegetarians in my office. Such a diet is worth a thought and, maybe, once in a while at least, worth giving a try. If you can't do it for your tastebuds, do it for your white blood cells. They work awfully hard, place themselves in danger's way, and like Rodney Dangerfield, they tend to get no respect.

Alternatively, another good way to protect ourselves from food industry harm is to make use of the Heart & Stroke Foundation of Canada's food information program, called Health Check (www.heartandstroke.com). Using the Canada Food Guide as a reference, each food product and restaurant dish in the Health Check program is evaluated by the Heart and Stroke Foundation's registered dieticians. Opting for food items in grocery stores and restaurants that display the Health Check symbol can help you choose foods that can be part of a healthy diet, and keep you away from the nasties that promote fat from depositing on your belly and cholesterol from depositing in your heart arteries.

Proof in the Pudding

If I were to choose one diet for its health benefits, sustainability, and tastiness, it would be— hands down— the Mediterranean Diet. While it may not be superior to others when it comes to weight loss, it is proven effective in reducing the risk of heart disease and stroke and is an easy diet to stick with. I know what you geography buffs are thinking: with over a dozen countries bordering the Mediterranean Sea, each with various cultural, ethnic, religious, and economic differences, how can there be a single Mediterranean Diet? Excellent question; and no, there isn't a single dietary regimen of the Mediterranean region. But there are some commonalities, which, as a whole, characterize the Mediterranean Diet (fig. 7.2).

Olive Oil is the predominant fat source
High consumption of fresh fruits, fresh vegetables, legumes, nuts and seeds
Moderate consumption of fish, poultry and dairy products
Low-to-moderate consumption of wine
Low consumption of red meat and eggs

Fig. 7.2 Mediterranean Diet Characteristics

The virtues of the Mediterranean Diet have been advocated in Europe since the Renaissance. In 1614, an exile from Modena, Italy, by the name of Giacomo Castelvetro, brought news of the Mediterranean Diet to Great Britain. After successfully fleeing the clutches of the Inquisition in Venice, he took refuge in Eltham, England and wrote a book entitled *The Fruit, Herbs and Vegetables of Italy*. He hoped to educate the backwards Brits about the importance of eating a wide variety of fruits and vegetables. Unfortunately, however, his book didn't take off during his lifetime. The publishing house never put the right kind of publicity behind his manuscript and his potential readership in Britain was far too enamored with their fried *Bubble and Squeak* to think fresh. "What's a matter for you?" Giacomo rightly asked, shaking his head, as the Brits avoided fruits and veggies and gorged themselves on meats and sweets.

The American physician, Ancel Keys, who developed the Minnesota Starvation Study discussed in Chapter Six, picked up where Giacomo had left off. While stationed in Salerno, Italy, he recognized that those living in the mountains of Crete had a lower incidence of heart disease and stroke than in other areas. "Could it be that these people are protected from cardiovascular disease because of the quantity of fruits and vegetables in their diet?" he wondered. To scientifically answer his question, he designed the landmark Seven Country Study. Over fifteen years, he studied dietary patterns and vascular disease prevalence in Greece and Italy, as well as Japan, Finland, the Netherlands, and the United States, for comparison.[190] His efforts were not wasted. The study showed a significant correlation between geographical location and cardiovascular disease, with the lowest rates of heart disease occurring in Greece and Italy. He was so convinced that it was indeed the Mediterranean style of diet that was responsible for the reduction in heart disease and stroke that he dedicated his remaining professional years to expounding the benefits of Mediterranean cooking concerning vascular disease prevention. And to really drive his point home, he lived to be 100 years of age. Now, that's walking the walk.

"That's very nice for those strolling along the Mediterranean Sea, but what about us North Americans? Can Dorothy and I benefit from eating such a diet, living in Kansas?" asks the Scarecrow of Dr. Oz.

As it turns out, it doesn't matter where those red pumps take you when you click your heels together—even no place but home—grub Med is good for you. The Lyon Heart Study demonstrated that even North Americans could reap significant cardiovascular health benefits by following a Mediterranean-style diet.[191] No matter if participants lived in Toronto or Tucson, shifting to a diet with higher amounts of fresh fruits and vegetables (at least 20 percent higher than our North American average) and a lower reliance on red meat consumption, significantly reduced the risk of vascular disease. "How significantly?" you ask. Well, buckle your seat belt, Dorothy, because this is going to knock your socks off! While following a Mediterranean-styled diet, the death rate in North American participants plummeted by an eye-popping 70 percent by comparison to those who persisted with their usual *Happy Meal* fare. The findings were so alarming that the ethics committee demanded the study be stopped, so the results could be made available to the public, without a moment to lose. And there still isn't a moment to lose. It's been shown more recently that even just substituting margarine, butter, mayonnaise, and dairy fat with olive oil can substantially lower the risk of cardiovascular disease.[192] So, ditch McDonald's, take your eyes off Wendy's, stop thinkin' Arby's, and embrace the Mediterranean style of eating—slow, fresh, and delightful, today!

United We Stand

Eating is risky behaviour; a moment on the lips and forever on your hips. And like other risky behaviours, such as alcohol consumption or sexual relations, we need to take intentional steps to protect ourselves from potential abuse. To prevent our appetites from taking on a life of their own, and to protect ourselves from over-eating or unhealthy eating, we are best to eat in community, together with family and friends. In addition to what Rudyard Kipling observed, that "He travels the fastest who travels alone," it's been demonstrated that he who eats alone, eats the fastest.[193] And it's not only speed; studies have shown that adults who eat alone are more likely to choose foods of higher fat content, particularly saturated fat, and eat fewer servings of fruit and vegetables.[194] The Binge Eating Disorder (BED) is a form of mental illness characterized by recurrent episodes of binge eating, where people suffer from loss of control over their food consumption.[195] They're often tormented by feelings of depression and guilt, eating when they're not hungry, and continuing to eat until they're uncomfortably full. One of the hallmarks of the Binge Eating Disorder is eating alone. Not surprisingly, one of the approaches to treating this disorder is to limit food intake to only times when two or more are gathered. The truth is this: we can all benefit from eating in community. For those following a diet plan, joining with others at mealtime can not only provide accountability for food choices and portion sizes but offer welcomed encouragement and support. So, just like the advice that Orson Welles received from his doctor, we should "stop having intimate dinners for four; unless there are three other people present."

Some years ago, my sister presented each of us, her siblings, with a handwritten collection of our mom's favourite recipes bound in a book: cinnamon pinwheels, currant scones, battered chicken. None of the recipes would catch Martha Stewart's attention, I'm sure, but they're *our* recipes. The book is filled with entrees and desserts that my siblings and I grew up with, and it means the world to us. My sister and her talented daughter individually annotated each recipe with stories and drawings that captured something of our family life, as we used to gather in the kitchen and eat together. It's a prized piece of work, more valuable to me than silver or gold because it speaks of my childhood memories in a way that no photo album or 16-mm movie film ever could. My eyes tear and my bottom lip sets to quivering every time I pull it off the shelf, but I continue to do so regularly, all the same. When I want to tell my boys a story from my youth, I spin the yarn over a dish from this collection. That way, they can taste and see how good it was.

The kitchen table is not only the primary place where we obtain our nutritional base; it's also the central location for fostering relationships and maintaining our cultural traditions. Around the kitchen table, we give and take, teach our children manners (and get reminded of a few ourselves), listen and are listened to, unpack our frustrating day at the office, encourage Johnny with his school project, sit, relax, celebrate, and let those pent-up stress hormones retreat a while. Consider the derivation of the word companion. It is two ancient words pasted together: "com" is Greek for "with" and "panis" is Latin for "bread." It follows, then, that our companions are those people with whom we break bread. We need these people. We can be most ourselves when we are in the company of those who know us best and in whom we can trust. Dorothy Day further defined companionship when she said, "Heaven is a banquet, and life is a banquet, too, even with a crust, where there is companionship." Perhaps, then, rather than reducing the mealtime to strictly chemicals and calories, believing "I am *what* I eat," we might consider the wealth of friendship and say, "I am *with whom* I eat." To optimize our health in the broadest sense of the word, we need to appreciate that our meals are as valuable as our medications, and recognize that our kitchens are at least as important a place as our diagnostic laboratories and medical clinics. We must guard against the destruction of hospitality and return the marginalized dinner meal from the sidelines and back to a central place in our lives. When we sit down to the dinner table with others and partake in a nutritional, healthy portioned meal together, we have the opportunity to not only cultivate friendships and traditions but vascular health as well.

Eating Ensemble

Two small towns in northern France illustrated the power of community in addressing the issue of obesity in school age children.[196] No, they didn't make a long-distance phone call to Jenny saying, "Excuse moi, Madame Craig, be sending us some of dis cuisine... Hors d'oeuvres, Cordon bleu, escargot and soupe du jour, s'il vous plaît... And don't scrimp on the pate, merci beaucoup!" Instead, the towns banded together in an all-out effort to encourage children to make healthy lifestyle choices, namely, eating nutritional food and increasing their activity levels. They enlisted the help of everyone in the community, from the schoolteachers, restaurant owners, caterers and shop owners, to the doctors, pharmacists, scientists, sport association leaders and media representatives. They even got the mayor and various branches of government to get up out of their chairs and take part in the esprit de corps. Together, they set up cooking workshops, funded dietary family counselling, built sporting facilities and playgrounds, developed walking and cycling routes, and hired sports instructors. After twelve years, the results were astounding—a real tour de force. The prevalence of overweight children had dropped to 8.8 percent, well below the neighbouring towns, where it had increased to the national average of nearly 18 percent. "C'est impressive," you say? That's exactly what the authorities said, and decided to extend the project to involve over 200 towns in Europe, under the name, EPODE (which stands for Ensemble, prevenons l'obésité des enfants, or Together, let's prevent obesity in children). We all need community, not only for sustainable weight loss and improved cardiovascular health but also for the joie de vivre!

Families Who Eat Together

"How about planning a family meal for the weekend?" I asked Marion. "That would be a step in health's direction for both you and your family."

"I suppose," she said tentatively, "but not without the television," she admitted. "I can't stop my grandkids from watching TV during dinner."

"Oh, sure you can," I argued. "Decorate the table with a nice tablecloth, light some candles, put on some music, and tell your family that it's a special night. Kids love celebrations," I said, undeterred by her negative vibes.

"And, what do I say that we're celebrating?" Marion

asked dryly, beginning to tire of my unsolicited advice.

"Be creative," I responded. "Make it a games night or choose a theme, like a Hawaiian Luau—my boys love to dress up. Or, just say that you're celebrating because it's Saturday—and it only comes once a week—and that you're all together, and you're all healthy... at least for the time being," I added after a deliberately long dramatic pause. "And, once you've established a regular weekend family meal, you can begin to plan weekday dinners, too."

"Well, like I said, with the busy lives we lead, that's just not practical," Marion started to remind me.

"Maybe it's not practical," I interjected, "but it's important. Making time for the family meal is a great way to not only foster healthy childhood development but safeguard our cardiovascular health into adulthood, as well. And it's not impossible, even with busy schedules. In our household, the slow cooker has helped address this 'too busy to do dinner' dilemma. We add the ingredients in the morning and, by the time we arrive home in the evening, dinner is hot and ready," I said.

"You mean that you use a crockpot?" Marion asked, scrunching up her face in disbelief. "I haven't seen those used for decades."

"Yeah, my mother tortured us kids with crockpot cooking, too," I agreed. "But, the slow cooker recipes have come a long way from those dark and dreary days. Check out *The Big Cook* cookbook, if you don't believe me. It was written by three busy moms who know all about hectic lifestyles and all about creative ways of putting the family meal on the table," I suggested, as I wrote out the book title on a prescription pad. "And if you want some other heart-healthy ideas, get a copy of Anne Lindsay's *New Lighthearted Cookbook*, or Bonnie Stern's *HeartSmart Cooking*."

"It's not that I don't want to," Marion explained, "it just seems like there's not enough time in the day."

"Yes, I agree. And, since time is precious, it might be an idea to look at Sandi Richard's *Cooking for the Rushed*. I don't do much more than look at the pictures myself, and peel potatoes and carrots, of course, but my wife swears by the recipes in these books. What they might lack in gourmet finesse, they make up for in a practical sense. And, what the world needs now is sense, sweet common sense."

Chapter Summary
Redefining Fine Dining

- Screen time, convenience foods, and busy time schedules have diminished the quantity and quality of family meals
- To avoid over-eating and consuming unhealthier fare, it's best not to mix screen time with snacks or mealtimes
- Yo-yo dieting can lower the basal metabolic rate and promote weight gain
- No one diet fits everyone

- Eating with others provides accountability, conversation, and is preferable to eating alone
- A sustainable healthy DIET should ideally be Diverse, Inexpensive, provide Essential nutrients, and be Timely (not too late in the evening)
- Fat-restricted diets have been shown to help slow vascular plaque progression and even assist regression of coronary artery disease
- The DASH diet is proven-effective for assisting blood pressure control
- Following the Mediterranean Diet is a sustainable and proven-effective approach to reduce cardiovascular disease
- Optimal weight control requires a long-range plan with permanent prudent dietary choices rather than following fad diets promising extravagant results
- Meal planning allows for healthier and more time-efficient options
- Prevention of obesity in our society is best accomplished with a multi-factorial community-based approach including dietary education, promotion of healthy eating habits, development of exercise programs and facilities, and the engagement of leadership

Chapter Notes

172. Shields M, Tremblay MS. Sedentary behaviour and obesity among Canadian adults. Health Reports (Statistics Canada, Catalogue 82-003) 2008; 19(2):19-30.

173. Fylan F, Harding GF. The effect of television frame rate on EEG abnormalities in photosensitive and pattern-sensitive epilepsy. Epilepsia. 1997 Oct;38(10):1124-31.

174. Zhuu W, Mantione K, Kream RM, Stefano GB. Alcohol-, nicotine-, and cocaine-evoked release of morphine from human white blood cells: substances of abuse actions converge on endogenous morphine release. Med Sci Monit. 2006 Nov;12(11):BR350-4.

175. Colapinto CK, Fitzgerald A, Taper LJ, Veugelers PJ. Children's preference for large portions: prevalence, determinants, and consequences. J Am Diet Assoc. 2007 Jul;107(7):1183-90.

176. Boutelle KN, Birnbaum AS, Lytle LA, Murray DM, Story M. Associations between perceived family meal environment and parent intake of fruit, vegetables, and fat. J Nutr Educ Behav. 2003 Jan-Feb;35(1):24-9.

177. Swinburn B, Shelly A. Effects of TV time and other sedentary pursuits. Int J Obes (Lond). 2008 Dec;32 Suppl 7:S132-6.

178. Veerman JL. By how much would limiting food advertising reduce childhood obesity? Eur J Public Health. Apr 14, 2009.

179. Touyz RM, Campbell N, Logan A, Gledhill N, Petrella R, Padwal R; Canadian Hypertension Education Program. The 2004 Canadian recommendations for the management of hypertension: Part III--Lifestyle modifications to prevent and control hypertension. Can J Cardiol. 2004 Jan;20(1):55-9.

180. American Heart Association Nutrition Committee, Lichtenstein AH, Appel LJ, Brands M, Carnethon M,

Daniels S, Franch HA, Franklin B, Kris-Etherton P, Harris WS, Howard B, Karanja N, Lefevre M, Rudel L, Sacks F, Van Horn L, Winston M, Wylie-Rosett J. Diet and lifestyle recommendations revision 2006: a scientific statement from the American Heart Association Nutrition Committee. Circulation. 2006 Jul 4;114(1):82-96.

181. Leung AK, Robson WL, Cho H, Lim SH. Latchkey children. J R Soc Health. 1996 Dec;116(6):356-9.

182. Martin Turcotte. The Time it Takes to Get to Work and Back. Statistics Canada 2005.

183. Resnick MD, Bearman PS, Blum RW, Bauman KE, Harris KM, Jones J, Tabor J, Beuhring T, Sieving RE, Shew M, Ireland M, Bearinger LH, Udry JR. Protecting adolescents from harm. Findings from the National Longitudinal Study on Adolescent Health. JAMA. 1997 Sep 10;278(10):823-32.

184. Burgess-Champoux TL, Larson N, Neumark-Sztainer D, Hannan PJ, Story M. Are family meal patterns associated with overall diet quality during the transition from early to middle adolescence? J Nutr Educ Behav. 2009 Mar-Apr;41(2):79-86.

185. Dansinger ML, Gleason JA, Griffith JL, Selker HP, Schaefer EJ. Comparison of the Atkins, Ornish, Weight Watchers, and Zone diets for weight loss and heart disease risk reduction: a randomized trial. JAMA 2005;293:43-53.

186. Sacks FM, Bray GA, Carey VJ, Smith SR, Ryan DH, Anton SD, McManus K, Champagne CM, Bishop LM, Laranjo N, Leboff MS, Rood JC, de Jonge L, Greenway FL, Loria CM, Obarzanek E, Williamson DA.Comparison of weight-loss diets with different compositions of fat, protein, and carbohydrates. N Engl J Med. 2009 Feb 26;360(9):859-73.

187. Lawes CM, Vander Hoorn S, Rodgers A. Global burden of blood pressure-related disease, 2001. Lancet 2008;371:1513-8.

188. Appel LM, Moore TJ, Obarzaneck E, et al. A clinical trial

of the effects of dietary patterns on blood pressure. N Engl J Med 1997;336:1117-24.

189. Ornish D, Sscherwitz LW, Billings JH. Intensive lifestyle changes for reversal of coronary heart disease. JAMA 1998;280(23):2001-2007.

190. Keys A. Coronary heart disease in seven countries. Circulation 1970;41 (Suppl 1):1-211.

191. de Lorgeril M, Salen P, Martin J. N. Mediterranean diet, traditional risk factors, and the rate of cardiovascular complications after myocardial infarction. Final report of the Lyon Diet Heart Study. Circ 1999;99(6):779-785.

192. Gutasch-Ferre, M et al. Olive oil consumption and cardiovascular risk in US Adults. J Am Coll Cardiol 2020; 75:1729-39.

193. Herman CP, Polivy J. Normative influences on food intake. Physiol Behav. 2005 Dec 15;86(5):762-72.

194. Larson NI, Nelson MC, Neumark-Sztainer D, Story M, Hannan PJ. Making time for meals: meal structure and associations with dietary intake in young adults. J Am Diet Assoc. 2009 Jan;109(1):72-9.

195. de Zwaan M. Binge eating disorder and obesity. Int J Obes Relat Metab Disord. 2001 May;25 Suppl 1:S51-5.

196. Romon M, Lommez A, Tafflet M. Basdevant A, Oppert JM, Bresson JL, Ducimetière P, Charles MA, Borys JM.Downward trends in the prevalence of childhood overweight in the setting of 12year school- and community-based programmes. Public Health Nutr 2008 December 23:1-8.

Chapter 8
Avoiding the After-Eight Mistake
Problems with Evening Calories

Eating Late Debate

"I just don't know why I can't lose any weight," Marion said, in an exasperated tone. "I'm walking most days now and I eat like a bird all day long!"

"It sounds frustrating," I empathized. "Tell me about it."

"I've been heavy most of my life," she went on. "There have only been two occasions when I was able to lose weight. One was when I was putting myself through college. I was a starving student back then—quite literally—and didn't have much money for basic groceries, let alone any goodies. And, the second time was during a six-week fast. I had protein shakes and water, and that's all," Marion explained.

"Neither sound like particularly healthy weight-loss strategies," I said.

"Oh, you're telling me. I don't ever want to see one of those protein drinks again!" she exclaimed. "It was dreadful. I felt awful and was tired all the time. But short of starving myself, I don't see how I can get rid of this," she complained, patting her abdomen.

"I'm no dietician," I admitted, "but why don't you walk me through a typical workday, and tell me what you usually eat. Maybe we can figure something out."

"Well, for starters... I still haven't got the breakfast thing figured out, and I know that's important, but I'm just too busy," she said, with a wave of her hand. "As for lunch... I've just been having a Caesar salad and maybe a bagel or scone," she explained.

"Sounds as if you're still a starving student," I smiled. "Don't you have anything else during the day?"

"Sure, I guess," she went on. "If someone brings baking into the office, I'll have something, and once in a while I eat a cookie or two—there's a big bag in the staff room, which is hard to ignore—and I usually have chocolate milk to wash them down. Sometimes, I have a couple Ultra Thin chocolates in the afternoon—but they're only 100 calories each, so they don't really count as anything."

"Seems as if you enjoy your sweet treats during the day. How about after dinner?" I asked.

"Yeah, after dinner, too," Marion said sheepishly. "If you really must know, I'm a bit of a late-night snacker," she confessed.

"That'll undo your daily walks in short order," I said. "You know Dr. Pamela Peeke's warning 'if you eat after eight, you'll gain a lot of weight,' right?"[197]

"Yes, I'm familiar with her books, but after dinner is the only time that I get to put my feet up for a while. Bill and I usually watch a little television, or if it's the weekend, we do some Netflix. I know that I should probably eat less in the evening, but that's when I'm most hungry," she said.

"Yes, and it's no wonder that you feel hungry in the evening," I agreed. "It sounds to me as if your body is trying to play catch-up after all that scrimping during the day. The type and timing of the calories we consume are as important as the amount," I added, and I turned over her electrocardiogram to draw a large triangle on the back of the page. "Since you're eating most of your calories in the evening, your daily calorie consumption is top-heavy and looks something like this," I said, holding up my triangle with the point directed downwards. "Weight control can often work better if we frontload our calories to provide our bodies with needed nutrients when they need them, starting with our morning breakfast, and then turn off calorie consumption in the evening," I said, rotating the page so the triangle peak pointed upwards. "In particular, we need to avoid late-night snacking with more in the morning, like the base of the triangle, and light at night, like the tip." (fig. 8.1).

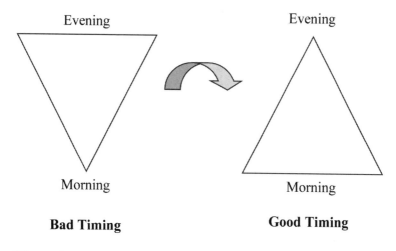

Figure 8.1 Optimizing Calorie Timing

"That may be true," Marion conceded. "But, I know full well that I'll still want something to eat in the evening. It's a habit I've gotten into. Don't you ever snack at night?" she asked imploringly.

"I might go through the motions of nibbling on something if we have company over, but generally, no, I don't snack after dinner. Instead, I usually make myself a pot of green tea in the evening. It's soothing to sip on, doesn't have any calories, and there's even some evidence that the polyphenols in green tea may help protect the heart and reduce dental caries—ticker and teeth, both."[198]

"No snacking at all?" Marion asked surprised. "Isn't that a bit severe? I mean, even Dr. Peeke says on her blog that you can have a small chocolate mousse bar before bed if you're hungry!"

"Not a chance. Chocolate mousse is the last thing you need in the evening and it will just end up on your thighs and abdomen," I warned. "We need to train our tastebuds not to expect stimulation after dinner, and to train our minds to prepare for needed rest, not repast."

Dieters in a Dangerous Time

The timing of food intake plays a significant role in weight control. As a general rule, evenly spaced calorie consumption is best, and earlier in the day is preferable to later. When it comes to evening, we need to be particularly careful to avoid eating. The hours between dinnertime and bedtime represent a veritable danger zone for dieters. Habitual nighttime eating is a recognized risk factor for the development of obesity. While evening snacking may be a common behaviour, it doesn't make it a healthy one. Studies have shown that, by contrast to those who snack at earlier times in the day, people who snack after dinner are more prone to weight gain.[199] This is because we're designed to be active and burn calories during the day and, then, rest and conserve our calories during the night. This phenomenon of variable calorie consumption is reflected in the diurnal pattern of stress hormone secretion. In the evening hours, as we wind down for the day, stress hormone levels also get turned down (fig. 8.2). As a result, calories ingested in the evening hours are less likely to be burned off and more likely to end up stored as fat. Elevated stress hormone levels in the morning may give us the green light to eat a nutritious breakfast, but the declining stress hormone levels in the evening necessitate that we put on the red light to nighttime snacking.

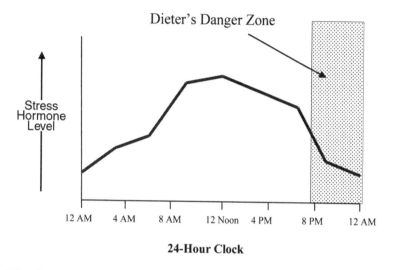

Fig. 8.2 Decline in Stress Hormones Mark the Dieter's Danger Zone

Dr. Albert Stunkard was one of the first to document this association between nighttime eating behaviour and the risk of obesity. He noted that people who ate during the evening— particularly, those who consumed more than 25 percent of their daily calories at night—had disrupted sleep patterns and ended up under-eating in the morning, perpetuating a bad cycle. In 1955, Stunkard dubbed the constellation of evening hyperphagia ("hyper" is "increased" and "phagia" is "eating"), morning anorexia, and sleep disturbances, the night eating syndrome (NES).[200] While there remains some controversy around the precise definition of NES, and whether or not it should be classified as a separate eating disorder, this much is generally agreed upon: like peanut butter and jelly or milk and cookies, NES and obesity go together. Obese patients are five times more likely to be diagnosed with NES than are normal-weight patients, and of patients being assessed for bariatric surgery, nearly 40 percent of them fit the criteria for NES.[201] Furthermore, people with NES have less success with weight loss and are more prone to weight regain.[202]

Repast Ruins Rhythm

Most of us have experienced the occasional disturbed sleep following a late-night eating fest. Heavy, spicy foods in particular, like curried lamb, jalapeño fajitas, or deep-fried wasabi chicken wings, are prone to mess with our slumber. However, for those who make a habit of noshing at night—even on healthy food choices—permanent disruptions in sleep patterns can ensue. It has to do with how our food consumption interacts with our natural biological clock, known as the circadian rhythm. Derived from the Latin words "circa" (around), and "diem" (day), the term circadian refers to events or things that span a full day, like waiting for a technical support operator on the 24-hour helpline. The circadian rhythm approximates the 24-hour day-night cycle and presides over many of our physiologic processes, including blood pressure control, digestive enzyme secretion, cortisol hormone levels, and our all-important sleep patterns. Our desire and ability to fall asleep is influenced by both the length of time we've been awake and by our internal circadian rhythms and explains why we are sleepy or wakeful at different times of the day.

Unlike my old Timex wristwatch, which takes a lickin' and keeps on tickin', our circadian clock needs continual adjustment and resetting. This is accomplished by several external time cues, referred to as *Zeitgebers* ("*zite*"-"gaybers") which is German for "time-givers." Like the studio producer who says "on in five," Zeitgebers act as a time reminder or prompt so we can be ready for "three, two, one, action!" These external stimuli provide the master clock in our brains with feedback to make fine adjustments to our circadian rhythm and keep our biological processes synchronized with one another, including energy balance, satiety signaling, and our cardiovascular function. While light exposure is the best-studied and most powerful Zeitgeber, it's not the only one. Other naturally occurring Zeitgebers include physical activity, ambient temperature, noise, and food consumption. Each of these factors works in conjunction with one another to synchronize our internal clock, reinforce our circadian rhythm, and establish our sleep/wake cycle. So, the problem with nighttime eating is this: making a habit of consuming calories in the evening sends the wrong message to our internal time-keeper, and confuses our sleep/wake cycle, producing measurable delays in the circadian rhythm. And here's the thing: circadian rhythm disruption has been shown to lead to weight gain.[203] It has to do with the satiety hormone leptin and its release into circulation. Discovered in 1994, leptin has been shown to be one of the key regulators of energy balance and, specifically, appetite regulation. Leptin signals our brains that we've had enough to eat and that we don't need that second smokie or third cupcake. Habitual nighttime eating affects leptin release. This may explain why those who eat in the evening, more often than not, are prone to struggle with weight gain.

Circadian Rhythm and Blues

Nighttime eating behaviour is not only associated with weight loss difficulties and obesity, it can be an indicator of deep-seated emotional distress. Although giving in to a late-night plate of mac 'n cheese or an occasional fudge brownie may not necessarily imply a melancholy mood, the habitual need to indulge in evening comfort food points towards trouble. There is a disease entity called Night Eating Syndrome (NES), which typically occurs in people with some form of psychosocial distress. Folks who suffer from NES end up disrupting their circadian rhythms resulting in a lowering of their levels of leptin and an increased risk of weight gain.[204] It's been demonstrated that those who are most susceptible to NES often suffer from depression, anxiety, anger, or poor social support and use food as a form of self-medication to gain comfort.[205] Whether the mood abnormalities initiate the night eating behaviour, or whether the night eating behaviour kicks off the mood abnormalities by way of circadian rhythm disruption, no one knows for sure. But, regardless of what comes first, NES and psychosocial distress go together like chickens and eggs. This is important to realize because psychosocial distress is a well-established risk factor for the development of premature heart disease and stroke.

The INTERHEART study group evaluated the relationship between stress and heart attack rates in their landmark worldwide study of cardiovascular risk factors. They defined stress as "feeling irritable, filled with anxiety, or as having sleeping difficulties as a result of conditions at work or at home." Their analysis demonstrated that the presence of stress ranked highly as a predictor of heart disease. In all fifty-two countries participating in the study, regardless of the age or gender of the participants, the same result was found: those who reported "permanent" stress either at home or their workplace had a twofold increased risk of suffering from a heart attack.[206] What's more, among those people with the highest levels of stress, there was a fourfold increase in the risk of cardiovascular death. The risk of stress-induced heart disease was found to have the same impact as smoking on our cardiovascular system and to carry almost twice the risk of high blood pressure.

Several screening tools have been developed to help us medics identify which of our patients may be suffering from psychosocial distress and which patients may benefit from more specific interventions, like targeted medications and professional counselling. Below is an example of a simple five-item questionnaire that we use to screen for depression, anxiety, anger and poor social support in our cardiology clinic (fig. 8.3).[207] A score of four or five is concerning, and a score over six in any one of the categories is a red flag, indicating the need for further assessment by a specialist. If you've got a tendency to overeat in the evening, psychosocial distress may be a root cause. Emotional eating is a common cause of obesity and weight-related issues. Read over the questionnaire and talk to your family physician about any high scores you identify.

Over the past two weeks, how much have you been bothered by _____?
Feeling sad, down, or uninterested in life?
Feeling anxious or nervous?
Feeling stressed?
Feeling angry?
Not having the social support you feel you need?

Fig. 8.3 STOP-D Screening Tool for Psychosocial Distress

Oral Interception

Psychosocial distress or not, nighttime eating is a formidable obstacle to losing extra weight. So, to optimize weight-reduction efforts, we must turn off calorie consumption in the evening. The following are some simple maneuvers that can help protect us from making the after-eight mistake of eating.

Snack-Proof Your House

You can't eat it if it's not there. Purging your pantry of fatty snacks like potato chips and cream puffs, salty fare like cheezies and pretzels, and sweet treats like chocolate bars and two-bite brownies removes the temptation to gorge if a late-night urge to eat strikes. A bare cupboard spared Old Mother Hubbard from over-feeding her doggie, and it can spare you, too, from unneeded calorie consumption and unwanted weight gain.

Just say 'No!' to Television

The invention of the television is listed by the National Academy of Engineering as one of the top twenty achievements of the 20th Century, right up there with the Model T Ford, Orville and Wilbur's magnificent flying machine and the indispensable Internet. And similar to other marvels of our modern era, television has promoted sedentary behaviour. The average North American adult watches fourteen hours of television per week and child watches twenty-five hours per week, with 20 percent of children watching forty-four hours![208] But, the relationship between television and obesity goes beyond the staggering number of hours that people sit glued in front of their flickering screens. It's all the potato chips, pretzels, nachos, ultra-thin wafers, Ritz crackers, and more that we consume while sitting on the sofa. Television is linked to obesity in part because we have linked watching television to food consumption.[209] This unhealthy marriage has not only fostered our obesity epidemic but threatens to accelerate the risk of heart disease and stroke, as well. Something's got to give. I suggest giving your diet a chance and giving up television.

Walk-a-Block

Going for a walk can not only help fill the time that might otherwise be devoted to snacking (especially in the early stages of changing our lifestyles), but it better prepares mind and body for sleep. And imagine: instead of consuming 200 more calories destined to join the fat stores around your middle, by walking smartly around the neighbourhood, you could *burn* 200 calories, and be that much closer to meeting both your fitness and weight-reduction goals. Weight management is more complex than the balance of energy input and energy output, but it certainly includes this simple equation, and we should take advantage of burning energy at every opportunity, the evening included.

Minty Freshness Prevents Fatness

Making an effort to clean your teeth right after dinner can be helpful with weight loss efforts. While brushing vigorously three times a day for two minutes at a time, could burn upwards of 3500 calories in a year (amounting to one pound of fat), the real benefits of brushing go far beyond whatever energy it consumes. When you brush your teeth after the dinner meal, you send a signal to your body that you're finished eating. Brushing with a strong peppermint toothpaste can distract your tastebuds long enough to allow your body time to register what food it's already eaten. Then, as levels of the hunger hormone, ghrelin, naturally fall off, satiety will be ushered in, diminishing your desire for a second helping. Careful flossing and rinsing can further thwart the craving for last-minute, unplanned, snacks, as you prepare for a good night's sleep. If you're dining out and don't want to carry your toothbrush along, consider packing some Listerine pocket strips. Their minty freshness is a real appetite killer. Try slipping one of those bad boys on your tongue after eating your dinner entree and see. The thought of having dessert will be far less appealing, if not downright revolting.

Clean Teeth Make for Clean Blood Vessels

As if derailing late-night snacking and giving weight loss efforts a fighting chance weren't reason enough to brush our teeth, there's a further health benefit that can be achieved by keeping our pearly whites pearly and white. No, I'm not referring to the reduced dental bills, the suspended nagging rebukes from your dental hygienist, nor to the silencing of your dentist's *tisk tisks* uttered as he taps over your molars like a colonel on the parade square. Regular brushing not only improves weight loss efforts, but it can also reduce the risk of heart disease and stroke. This link between teeth and ticker is a bit complex, but it's well worth appreciating, especially if you're worried enough about your heart health to buy a book on the subject like this one. So, bear with me for a few paragraphs, if you will, and let me try to explain just how clean teeth can help us maintain clean blood vessels.

To understand how dental health can affect heart health, it's important to appreciate that the hordes of bacteria bustling about in our mouths aren't just sitting idly by and twiddling their thumbs. Rather, those little beasties are hell-bent on destruction! The wee microbial monsters infect our gums, strip the enamel from our teeth, rot their roots and, in the process, stir up our inflammatory machinery, which can wreak havoc in our bloodstreams. Oral bacteria are so destructive because they convert dietary sugars, like those so abundantly supplied at the snack bar, into acidic waste products. When mixed in with our saliva, the acid acts like a corrosive bath in which our teeth and gums bathe. And, regardless of what Madge might say, we shouldn't relax as we soak in it! Although it's a relatively mild acid, we don't want our teeth soaking in it for prolonged periods. The acidic environment not only contributes to our less than appealing gorilla breath, but it also dissolves our dental enamel, weakens and discolors our teeth, and leads to dental caries (cavities). As well, the bacterial toxins irritate our gums, causing them to become red, swollen and inflamed, a phenomenon called gingivitis ("gingiva" is Latin for "gums" and "itis" refers to inflammation). And here's the real concern: both dental caries and gingivitis give bacteria and their toxic waste products access to our cardiovascular system. It's been shown that bacterial toxins can gain access to our bloodstream via damaged teeth and across diseased gums and accelerate plaque formation within the walls of our blood vessels (fig. 8.4).[210]

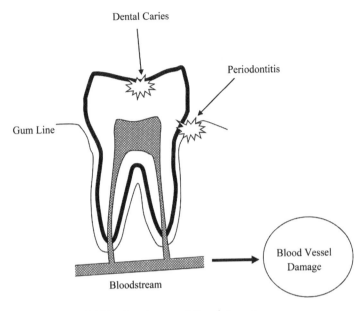

Fig. 8.4 Bacterial Toxins Access Bloodstream

Allowing bacteria to flourish in our mouths increases the likelihood that their toxic byproducts will accumulate and then spill into our bloodstream. The bacterial toxins that leak into our bloodstream from our mouths turn on our inflammatory machinery. Our immune system responds to the mess of bacterial toxins by increasing the numbers of patrolling white blood cells that circulate through our bodies to clean them up. In the process, however, the increased activity of our immune system inadvertently damages the endothelial cells that line our blood vessels. Over time, this endothelial injury can accelerate vascular plaque formation and take us down the dark and dreary road to atherosclerosis. In this way then, dental plaques can beget vascular plaques, and increase our risk of heart disease and stroke.

To see if gum disease is already at work in your mouth, turn up the vanity lights in your bathroom and take a close look at your mouth in the mirror. The gum tissue next to your teeth should be light pink, like the color of a Salmon Crayola Crayon, blanching with pressure from your finger. When our gums get inflamed, however, this tooth/tissue interface becomes reddened like a Hot Magenta crayon and is prone to bleeding. Over time, persistent inflammation around our gums causes the gums to recede, exposing previously covered enamel to the scourge of bacterial acidic waste. And, just as recession is hard on the economy and your investment broker's hairline, it's also detrimental to dental health. As our protecting gums get infected and recede, bacteria can form gingival pockets below the gum line and penetrate farther down between our teeth and gums, invading the deeper tissue layers. Inflammation of the supporting tissues around our teeth is termed periodontitis ("peri" means "around," "odont" refers to "tooth," and "itis" indicates "inflammation"). Bacterial toxins, as well as our body's enzymes released from white blood cells quelling the toxic attack, can break down the surrounding bone and connective tissues that hold teeth in place. Too much of this sport eventually leads to tooth loss. Don't fool yourself; it could happen to you. As well, people with gum disease not only have higher levels of inflammation in their mouths, but they also have more inflammation going on in their bloodstreams, with elevated CRP levels to prove it. And where there's an elevated CRP level, there's an increased risk of cardiovascular catastrophe.[211]

Put Some Muscle Where Your Mouth Is

The tooth/ticker story doesn't have to end sadly. With some attention to improved dental hygiene, the inflammation that bacteria produce in our mouths and the systemic inflammation in our bloodstreams that follows can be significantly diminished. Even if our gums and teeth have been beaten up and battered over the years, dental health can be reclaimed if we begin to handle our mouths with care. It's been demonstrated that when people with inflamed gums and high CRP levels undergo regular professional dental cleaning, gingivitis resolves, inflammation settles, and CRP levels return to normal.[212]

Regular biannual dental review can address tooth decay issues and help keep gum disease in check. Professional plaque removal is a proven effective strategy to both improve dental health and reduce the inflammation in our blood vessel walls.[213] Dental hygienists are best able to remove stubborn and hard-to-reach dental plaques by a process called scaling. This expert cleaning of tooth surfaces helps to destabilize bacterial footholds and reduce the likelihood that bacterial toxins spill into our circulation. Periodontal therapy has been shown to enhance healthy tooth surfaces, and reduce attachment loss, allowing our teeth to stay where they belong—in our mouths chewing. Serial x-rays can allow dentists to better assess areas of oral discomfort and estimate the amount of bone loss between and around the teeth. Dentists also make a habit of inspecting the tongue, cheeks, and throat for early signs of oral cancer, particularly important for the resolute smokers in the crowd. It's ideal to attend the same dental clinic, where your dental records and x-rays can be reviewed as needed. Your dentist is then in the best position to assess your dental hygiene progress over time and can help develop a staged intervention plan to optimize your oral health and, indirectly, enhance your cardiovascular health. If we're serious about reducing the risk of heart disease and stroke, making an appointment with a dentist is an excellent starting place.

Dental health is too important to only address every nine to twelve months with professional cleaning. Fighting dental plaque is everyone's battle. We each need to take some responsibility for our health and our teeth are an excellent starting place. The important work of dentists and dental hygienists needs to be complemented by our close attention to oral care at home. A daily, three-step dental hygiene approach of brushing, flossing, and rinsing can effectively reduce bacterial plaque buildup and help intercept oral inflammation before it causes vascular inflammation.

Step 1. Don't Rush, Brush

Add "new toothbrush" to the top of your shopping list.

When used properly, and not just left neglected in a cup on the counter, toothbrushes get a lot of wear and tear. It's recommended that we replace our toothbrush every three months, and c'mon, now, let's be honest; it's been more than three months since you've replaced that ratty old toothbrush of yours with the matted bristles and faded handle (Wasn't that the one that was included in your Y2K emergency kit?). Using a brush with medium to soft bristles helps minimize gum trauma, as does brushing with a little tenderness. Gum inflammation can be reduced by applying the sides of the bristles against the gums with a gentle massaging action of the brush to stimulate them, not a sawing action to mutilate them. For a little excitement, consider purchasing a vibrating tool—an electric toothbrush that is. Adding an electric toothbrush to your dental armamentarium can complement manual brushing efforts and improve cleaning thoroughness, and the expense pays dividends at the dentist's office. Using a fluoride toothpaste helps to strengthen tooth enamel and protect it from the damaging effects of bacterial acid. Remineralization of the tooth enamel is a dynamic process, and fluoride from toothpaste is incorporated into the enamel on exposure, making teeth less vulnerable to bacterial attack.

A useful exercise to check your brushing technique is to use plaque disclosing tablets. The school nurse used to hand out the red dye pills to us elementary school kids during Dental Week, to illustrate the need for careful brushing. First, we were asked to brush in our usual manner. Then, we were asked to chew on a dye pill and swish the accumulated saliva around in our mouths for about a minute. In addition to turning our tongues bright scarlet, the red chemical attached to areas of dental plaque on our teeth and demonstrated where we needed to give more attention. Even as a child, it was a very humbling experience to smile in front of the mirror after having just brushed madly and see a mouthful of red-stained teeth.

While the verdict is still out on how often we should brush our teeth—once, twice, three times a day—for optimal oral care, each tooth surface needs to be carefully scrubbed at least once a day to remove food debris and bacteria. I usually do a cursory brushing first thing in the morning to freshen my breath. Since nearly half of oral bacteria lurk amid our 3000 taste receptors, to improve my chances of taming my jungle breath, I make sure to brush my tongue surface, as well. Then, I brush my teeth again, before seeing patients in my clinic, to get rid of the garlic odor on my breath and any adherent pieces of parsley left from lunch. But, my main attack on plaque is in the evening. Before retiring for bed, I've usually got more time to do a thorough job of cleaning my teeth, and I'm less prone to slovenly rush n' brush. As well, saliva production is reduced during our sleeping hours. This is important to know since saliva helps to protect our mouths, washing over our teeth and gums, and flushing oral bacteria down to a stomach acid watery grave.[214] At night, the flow from our salivary glands decreases, and there's less saliva to combat bacteria and offset the caustic effects of their toxic by-products on our mouths. With less spit defending our teeth during the wee hours, it makes sense to polish them well before sleeping. That way, as we settle into our beds and grab some shut-eye, bacteria are less apt to settle into our gums and grab a foothold.

Step 2. Floss the Dross

Set aside a few minutes every evening to give the bacteria in your mouth their walking papers: floss them out of house and home. Brushing is a good start towards improved dental hygiene, but without flossing it's only a half job. Carefully flossing around both sides of each tooth removes the bacterial biofilm collected over the day and helps to more effectively reduce plaque accumulation and tooth discoloration. My wife is so proficient at cleaning her teeth that she can floss while supervising our teen's math homework. My teeth, however, are quite crowded, so flossing has always been a bit of a chore for me, requiring my undivided attention. I don't go at it like Tom Hanks did in the movie *Turner and Hooch*, where he used a separate piece of dental floss for each tooth. Instead, I tear off a little more than half a metre, or about eighteen inches, of dental floss to tackle the job, unless the floss gets stuck between my teeth and breaks during attempts to free it. I've been told that in troublesome areas I'm supposed to just let go of one end of the floss and pull it out the other side, but thanks to wax-coated floss or dental tape, the slide action has made my flossing attempts easier.

"Flossing does two things for me pretty consistently," I complained to my dental hygienist during one of her lengthy reprimands. "It cuts off the circulation to my fingers making the tips turn white and the pads numb, and it makes my gums bleed."

"With proper technique," she explained to me patiently, "flossing reduces dental plaque buildup more effectively than brushing can alone. Try wrapping the dental floss around your middle two fingers on each hand and then manipulate the floss with your index fingers for your upper teeth, and your thumbs for your lower teeth. The more regularly one flosses, the less bleeding occurs and the less painful a process it becomes."

"But flossing is such a great big bore," I went on. "Is it absolutely critical to floss around every single tooth, every single day?"

"Oh, no, not at all," she said, with a smile. "Just floss around the teeth you want to keep."

Step 3. Rinse for the Glints

Swish, swash, or spit, but don't just leave food debris and bacteria hanging there on your teeth after eating. Although the glory days of the spittoon are long passed, the importance of great expectorations is not. To most effectively reduce oral bacteria numbers, we need to rinse our mouths thoroughly after meals and snacks. Using mouthwash may seem like good money down the drain, but my dental colleagues disagree. They say that the use of an antimicrobial mouth rinse immediately after flossing helps to delay the recolonization of bacteria on the freshly cleaned tooth surfaces and may assist in improving oral health.[215] Since prolonged mouthwash exposure can damage the oral mucosa, there's no need to hold the rinse in your mouth for any longer than the few seconds it takes to swish it about your mouth. It is a good idea to rinse your mouth at some point after you've flossed your teeth so that the loosened debris exits your mouth. Daily use of chlorhexidine mouth rinse following mechanical brushing and flossing care has been shown to effectively reduce dental staining and plaque formation.[216]

Carpe P.M.

"Brushing your teeth after dinner and purging the pantry of junk food will help reduce the temptation to eat empty calories in the evening hours," I said to Marion, "but, it's also important to refrain from *drinking* empty calories, too."

"Yes, that's why I drink more diet pop these days," Marion said in agreement.

"Good, but how about alcohol; how much happy juice do you drink?" I asked point-blank, keeping in mind, of course, that we all tend to underestimate how much alcohol we consume.

"Oh, not much," she offered. "One or two drinks a day, perhaps, mainly on the weekends, and when we have friends over. There's nothing wrong with that, is there?'"

"Having friends over? No. Not at all," I replied with a smile, "but maybe with the amount of booze."

"But I thought that a couple of drinks were good for the ticker," Marion countered, tapping her chest. "Bill's always going on about how the antioxidants in his wine are so 'good for the heart.' Isn't that right?"

"Sure, red wine contains bioflavonoids, phenolics, resveratrol, and other anti-oxidant constituents which may offer some vascular protection," I agreed, "similar to unfermented grape juice and raisins, actually. But, despite what the wine industry might say, the most beneficial ingredient in alcohol is the alcohol itself, or, to be more precise, the ethanol, when consumed in the range of 20 to 30 grams per day. The mechanism is complex and involves alcohol's positive influence on a variety of heart-health parameters, including reducing inflammation and blood-clotting proteins, and raising insulin sensitivity and good cholesterol levels."[217]

"So, wine, beer, or a good ol' G&T, it doesn't matter the type of drink?" Marion asked, delighted to have one over on her husband.

"Yes, so long as you don't drink too much," I cautioned. "Alcohol has a narrow therapeutic window. The mortality curve is J-shaped,[218] and looks a bit like the Nike swoosh symbol," I said, motioning with my hand in the air (fig. 8.5). "Anything more than one or two drinks per day and the health benefits quickly fall away. At higher than mild to moderate doses, alcohol is toxic and can cause high blood pressure, heart rhythm disorders, heart failure, and even sudden cardiac death, not to mention cirrhosis of the liver."[219]

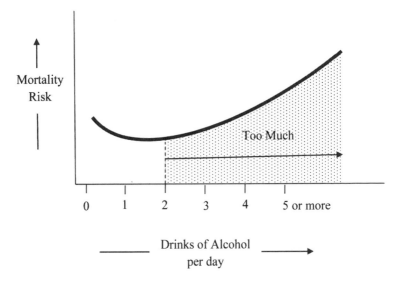

Fig. 8.5 J-Shaped "Swoosh" Curve of Alcohol Consumption and Mortality Risk

"But, one or two drinks are still okay for me to have once in a while?" asked Marion.

"Not if losing weight is on your 'to-do' list," I replied, shaking my head. "It's important to remember that drinking alcohol is fattening and mixed drinks, in particular, contain far too many empty calories (table 8.1).[220] If you're serious about losing weight, then alcohol needs to be off-limits, in the same way cheesecake and poutine are verboten. For those people who have attained their ideal body weight and follow a healthy lifestyle, including daily exercise, a glass of wine or a shot of port may be fine, now and again, and perhaps even advantageous.[221] But, if you're struggling with weight gain, then water should be your main beverage."

Alcoholic Beverage	Empty Calories
One ounce of 80-proof alcohol	90
Glass of white wine (140 ml or 5 fluid oz)	110
Glass of red wine (140 ml or 5 fluid oz)	120
Bottle of beer (341 ml at 5% alcohol)	150
Bottle of 'light' beer	116
Bailey's Irish Cream (2.5 ounces)	170
Gin and Tonic	200
Mai Tai	350
White Russian	425
Pina Colada	644
Margarita	740
Long Island Ice Tea	780

Table 8.1 Calorie Content in Selected Alcoholic Beverages

"Well, it's not that I *need* the alcohol," Marion said honestly. "But, it's hard to have just plain water when everyone else is having a special drink. I don't want to be anti-social."

"Anti-social or not, I still think that water should be our number one source of hydration," I argued, "Especially if weight management is your concern. However, if you want to join the fray, then consider tonic water minus the gin, or even better, sparkling mineral water. To liven it up a bit, throw in some fruit juice ice cubes or a lemon wedge. And think of it this way: when your friends raise their glasses to toast their health, at least your *non-alcoholic* drink will be healthier."

"I suppose," Marion conceded. "But, it doesn't sound very fun or very relaxing for that matter. After a long day, I need to relax. A glass of wine, as I sit down to a favourite program on Crave, helps me do that."

Relaxing in the evenings is very important for all of us," I agreed. "But, alcohol doesn't need be part of that equation. And, you've got better things to do with your precious evening hours than waste them watching television. I'd suggest putting a cap on the nightcap, turning off the television, shutting down the computer, and using the time in the evening to prepare for tomorrow; you know, set up for breakfast, make lunch, and lay out your clothing for the next day."

"Oh, you're just trying to get me organized," Marion protested.

"Absolutely," I agreed with a smile, "and, of course, I want to help you reduce your waistline and your risk of developing heart disease. The evening is an opportunity for building health; so, we need to seize it. Let me tell you how I relax come nightfall," I said, as I grabbed one of my prescription pads to write on. "First off, I *Rinse* my mouth right after dinner and brush my teeth with minty toothpaste to kill any desire for dessert or other late-night snacks; I *Eat* nothing in the evening; I *Listen* to some quiet music as I get things organized for the morning; I *Avoid* alcohol; and I spend time with my boys reading a book, *eXchanging* it for watching television. Then, to get drowsy, I settle into bed with one of my medical journals, and I'm out like a light. If you can relax in these sorts of ways," I added, handing her the prescription sheet I was writing on (fig. 8.6), "you'll struggle far less with weight gain and be making important strides forward on the health highway during the evening hours."

R

- **R**inse your mouth
- **E**at nothing
- **L**isten to music
- **A**bstain from alcohol
- **X**-change TV for reading

Fig. 8.6 Evening Prescription to Relax

Chapter Summary
Avoiding the After Eight Mistake

- Calorie consumption for the day should follow the shape of a pyramid, more in the morning, less in the evening

- The hours between dinnertime and bedtime represent a veritable danger zone for dieters
- Late-night snacking can upset our circadian rhythms and lead to weight gain
- Levels of the satiety hormone leptin are reduced with evening snacking
- Levels of the hunger hormone ghrelin are elevated with evening snacking
- STOP-D Screening Tool can help identify people with emotional eating habits related to psychosocial distress
- Snack-proofing your house can help reduce evening junk food binging
- Attention to proper dental hygiene in the form of regular brushing, flossing, and rinsing can help reduce vascular inflammation and improve cardiovascular health

- Alcohol contains only empty calories and should be avoided if weight loss is desired

- RELAX prescription: Rinse; Eat nothing; Listen to music; Avoid alcohol; eXchange screen time for an evening walk or reading a book

Chapter Notes

197. Pamela Peek. Fight Fat After Forty, Viking Penguin 2000.

198. Ghosh D, Scheepens A. Vascular action of polyphenols. Mol Nutr Food Res. 2009 Mar;53(3):322-31.

199. Gluck ME, Venti CA, Salbe AD, Krakoff J. Nighttime eating: commonly observed and related to weight gain in an inpatient food intake study. Am J Clin Nutr 2008;88(4):900-905.

200. Stunkard AG, Grace WJ, Wolff HG. The night-eating syndrome; a pattern of food intake among certain obese patients. Am J Med 1955;19:78-

201. Allison KC, Wadden TA, Sarwer DB, et al. Night eating syndrome and binge eating disorder among persons seeking bariatric surgery: prevalence and related features. Surg Obes Relat Dis 2006;2:153–8.

202. Powers PS, Perez A, Boyd F, Rosemurgy A. Eating pathology before and after bariatric surgery: a prospective study. Int J Eat Dis 1999;25:293-300.

203. Arble D, Bass J, Laposky AD, Vitaterna MH, Turek FW. Circadian timing of food intake contributes to weight gain. Obesity 2009;17(11):2100-2102.

204. Goel N, Stunkard AJ, Rogers NL, Van Dongen HP, et al. Circadian rhythm profiles in women with night eating syndrome. J Biol Rhythms. 2009 Feb;24(1):85-94.

205. Caredda M, Roscioli C, Mistretta M, Pacitti F. Stress vulnerability and night eating syndrome in the general population. Riv Psichiatr 2009 Jan-Feb;44(1):45-54.

206. Rosengren A, Hawken S, Ounpuu S, et al. Association of psychosocial risk factors with risk of acute myocardial infarction in 11,119 cases and 13,646 controls from 52 countries (the INTERHEART study): case-control study. Lancet 2004;364:953-62.

207. Young QR, Ignaszewski A, Fofonoff D, et al. Brief screen to identify 5 most common forms of psychosocial distress in cardiac patients: validation of the screening tool for psychosocial distress (STOP-D). J Cardiovasc Nursing 2007;22:525-34

208. Gentile DA, Walsh DA. A normative study of family media habits. Applied Developmental Psychology 2002;23:157-178.

209. Thomson M, Spence JC, Raine K, Laing L. The association of television viewing with snacking behavior and bodyweight of young adults. Am J Health Promot. 2008 May-Jun;22(5):329-35.

210. Douglass CW. Risk assessment and management of periodontal disease. J Am Dent Assoc 2006;137(suppl 3):27S-32S.

211. Ridker PM, Rifai N, Rose L, Buring JE, Cook NR. Comparison of C-reactive protein and low density lipoprotein cholesterol levels in the prediction of first cardiovascular events. N Engl J Med. 2002 Nov 14;347(20):1557-65.

212. Tonetti MS, D'Aiuto F, Nibali L, Donald A, Storry C, Parkar M, Suvan J, Hingorani AD, Vallance P, Deanfield J. Treatment of periodontitis and endothelial function. N Engl J Med. 2007 Mar 1;356(9):911-20.

213. Douglass CW. Risk assessment and management of periodontal disease. J Am Dent Assoc 2006;137(suppl 3):27S-32S.

214. The role of saliva in maintaining oral health and as an aid to diagnosis. Med Oral Patol Oral Cir Bucal. 2006 Aug;11(5):E449-455.

215. Kolahi J, Soolari A. Rinsing with chlorhexidine gluconate solution after brushing and flossing teeth: a systematic review of effectiveness. Quintessence Int. 2006 Sept;37(8):605-612.

216. Barnett ML. The rationale for the daily use of an

antimicrobial mouthrinse. J Am Dent Assoc. 2006 Nov;137 Suppl 3:16S-21S.

217. Mukamal KJ, Jensen MK, Gronbaek M. Drinking frequency mediating biomarkers and risk of myocardial infaction in women and men. Circulation 2005;112:1406-13.

218. DiCastelnuovo A, Casatanzo S, Bagnardi V, et al. Alcohol dosing and total mortality in men and women. Arch Intern Med 2006;166:2437-45.

219. Fenske, TK. Alcohol and the Heart: a look at both sides. Perspectives in Cardiology, May 2008;24(5):27-30.

220. Dorn JM, Hovey K, Muti P, et al. Alcohol drinking patterns differentially affect central adiposity as measured by abdominal height in women and men. J Nutr 2003;133:2655-62.

221. Mukamal KJ, Chiuve SE, Rimm EB. Alcohol consumption and risk for coronary heart disease in men with healthy lifestyles. Arch Intern Med 2006;166:2145-50.

Chapter 9
The Beauty of Rest
Health Benefits of Sleep

Weight Loss Obstructions

"Of course, it's not all just attention to diet and exercise," I explained to Marion. "There are many medical conditions that can significantly undermine weight loss efforts."

"Oh, like glandular disorders?" she interjected. "I've heard about those and I've often felt that I must have one."

"No, that's not what I was referring to," I said, restarting my train of thought. "There are several biological disorders, such as clinical depression, obstructive sleep apnea, and ADHD that can make losing weight doubly difficult."

"ADHD?" Marion asked, perplexed. "You mean adults can get *Attention-Deficit/Hyperactivity Disorder*, too? That's what my eldest granddaughter has, and it drives my daughter nuts... although things have improved, somewhat, since she's been on Ritalin."

"Yes, ADHD is not just a childhood disease," I explained. "Although it's more common in school-age children, symptoms of inattention, hyperactivity and impulsivity can persist into adulthood. ADHD is one of the most common chronic psychiatric disorders occurring in adults. It's been estimated that 5 percent of adults in the general population have Attention Deficit, and the proportion is considerably higher among those with obesity (fig. 9.1).[222] And sadly, ADHD often goes undiagnosed in adults."[223]

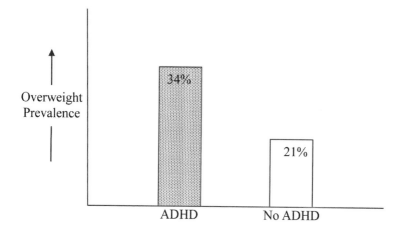

Fig. 9.1 Higher Prevalence of Obesity/Overweight in ADHD group than in people without ADHD[224]

"Really?" Marion asked, quite surprised. "How do you make the diagnosis of Attention Deficit in adults?"

"Well... I don't. I leave the diagnosis of ADHD to the professionals. But, I do use this screening quiz, from time to time, that can help identify patients prone to ADHD," I said, handing Marion a photocopy of the World Health Organization Adult ADHD Self-Report Scale (table 9.1).[225] "A score of 11 points or higher is suggestive of Adult Attention-Deficit/Hyperactivity Disorder, and warrants further evaluation by your family doctor."

Circle the number that best describes how you have felt or conducted yourself over the past six months	Never	Rarely	Sometimes	Often	Very Often	Score
How often do you have trouble wrapping up the final details of a project once the challenging parts have been done?	0	1	2	3	4	
How often do you have difficulty getting things in order when you have to do an organizational task?	0	1	2	3	4	
How often do you have problems remembering appointments or obligations?	0	1	2	3	4	
How often do you delay getting started on a task that requires a lot of thought?	0	1	2	3	4	
How often do you fidget or squirm with your hands or feet when you have to sit for a long time?	0	1	2	3	4	
How often do you feel overly active and compelled to do things like you were driven by a motor?	0	1	2	3	4	
In people aged 18 years or older, a score of 11 points or higher suggests the diagnosis of Adult ADHD and that it may be beneficial to undergo further evaluation by your healthcare provider	Total					

Table 9.1 Adult ADHD Screening Questionnaire[226]

"Why is ADHD more common in people who are

overweight?" Marion asked as she looked over the questionnaire.

"Oh... theories abound," I sighed. "Some people think that the symptoms of ADHD are related to excessive television and computer use, suggesting that such activities rewire our brains and make us more impulsive.[227] Binge eating is a prime example of impulsive behaviour and could certainly contribute to obesity in ADHD patients. As well, sleep deprivation may be part of the reason why there is such an overlap between ADHD and obesity. ADHD behaviours have been shown to be related to insufficient sleep, and so has weight gain."[228]

"Well, I think my attention span is probably okay," Marion said, as she put the questionnaire back on the table. "But I certainly don't sleep well. It doesn't help matters, I suppose, that my husband, Bill, has sleep apnea."

"He's a bit of a snorer at night, is he?" I asked, empathetically.

"Bit of a snorer?!" she exclaimed. "He sounds more like a sawmill!"

"But, doesn't he have a CPAP (continuous positive airway pressure) machine to help him breathe properly at night?" I asked.

"Yes, he has a machine, and he did use it... at least initially," she explained. "But he's been having some difficulty getting a mask that fits his face properly—one leaks air, the other is too tight—and he claims that the airflow makes his nasal congestion worse and gives him claustrophobia. He's a really difficult one to please," Marion said in a sing-song voice while shaking her head. "And, after thirty-two years of marriage, I should know."

"I think it would be important for him to be reviewed by the pulmonary team to get those issues properly addressed," I emphasized. "Obstructive sleep apnea is very treatable these days and treatment has been shown to not only improve sleep quality, but also reduce the risks of heart disease and stroke, and even improve weight control efforts."[229]

"Weight control?" Marion asked, puzzled. "I've heard that losing weight can improve sleep apnea, but I didn't know that treatment of sleep apnea could help with losing weight."

"Yes, they both go hand in hand," I explained. "Inadequate sleep interferes with daytime alertness, depletes energy levels, and places people in a poor position to follow through with a prudent diet or being physically active. And while treatment of sleep apnea isn't a standalone solution for losing weight, regular use of CPAP in overweight patients with obstructive sleep apnea has been shown to improve a variety of metabolic parameters and facilitate weight loss."[230]

Snooze To Lose

I hate to miss out on a good night's sleep. It makes me irritable, impatient, foggy in the head, and inexorably fatigued. And if my sleep deprivation gets prolonged, as when I take my turn providing nighttime coverage of the coronary care unit over a weekend, I predictably come down with post-nasal drip, a sore throat, and a whopper of a headache. It doesn't surprise me to learn that sleep deprivation has been used in torture chambers and during prisoner interrogation; it's downright painful. The former Prime Minister of Israel, Menachem Begin, became familiar with this type of suffering as a prisoner of the KGB during WWII. In recounting his experience of forced sleep deprivation, he described that "In the head of the interrogated prisoner, a haze begins to form. His spirit is wearied to death, his legs are unsteady, and he has one sole desire: to sleep. Anyone who has experienced this desire knows that not even hunger and thirst are comparable with it."[231] There's no doubt that extended sleep deprivation can be stressful on the mind, body, and soul. But it's important to realize that we don't have to be in the extreme state of hazy thoughts and unsteady legs to suffer from lack of sleep; even mild degrees of sleep deprivation can be detrimental to our wellbeing. When we stay up late to watch the *Late Show* or rise early to beat the rush hour, we are subjecting our bodies to the harmful effects of stress and robbing ourselves of an opportunity to build health.

While many aspects about sleep remain a mystery to modern science, investigations have consistently shown that restorative sleep plays a central role in a wide variety of bodily functions, from the intellectual arena of problem-solving ability and memory consolidation to the physical realm of muscle growth, hormonal balance, and the maintenance of our immune system. Our cardiovascular system also needs proper amounts of quality sleep for optimal function. When we sleep, we enter a hibernation-like state: our heart rate and respiration slow, blood pressure falls, and our body core temperature drops. Since the workload for our heart is directly related to both the heart rate and blood pressure, slumber brings relative reprieve for our persistently pumping heart muscles. But the benefits of sleep for the heart are more deep-seated than mere energy management. Sleep brings restoration to our blood vessels, without which the day's damages can develop into disease. It is during our sleeping hours that the lining of our vasculature gets revitalized.[232] The injuries suffered by our blood vessel linings from the day's combat, like skipping breakfast, eating that double chocolate doughnut during a coffee break, or battling through downtown traffic, are repaired and smoothed over by the work of specialized, white blood cells while we sleep. What's more, sleep allows our vascular cells to reinforce their armor in preparation for the next day's cellular battle. The cells that make up our vascular lining produce nitric oxide, which functions to protect our blood vessels from the wear and tear of daily stressors. As we sleep, our stores of nitric oxide are replenished, making our vascular lining less susceptible to injury. William Shakespeare may not have known about the many physiological benefits of restorative sleep, but he hinted at them eloquently in *Macbeth* when he wrote, "Sleep that knits up the ravelled sleeve of care / The death of each day's life, sore labour's bath / Balm of hurt minds, great nature's second course, / Chief nourisher in life's feast."[233]

The restoration that occurs as we sleep is nourishment for our body and soul. It gives us a "second course" which adds no calories, and a "feast" which produces no waistline gain.

When we don't get the sleep we need, our bodies respond by secreting the stress hormone cortisol into our bloodstream, in the hopes that this may somehow help. But, of course, this doesn't, and just the opposite occurs. Stress hormones may help us prepare for the fight of the day, but as evening draws nigh, elevated cortisol levels are counterproductive to sleeping. We may be able to readily recover from transient cortisol elevations following an isolated all-nighter in the office or from an occasional trans-Atlantic plane flight, but persistent cortisol elevations aren't so easy to shake. Chronic sleep deprivation sets in motion a downward spiral of sleep disruption. As a result, the less we sleep, the less we *can* sleep. This is because cortisol secretion is normally under what's called negative feedback control. It's a common control mechanism for hormonal activity, and similar to the thermostat in a house. Just as the thermostat turns the furnace off when the desired room temperature has been reached, so, too, transiently elevated cortisol levels send a message back to the adrenal glands (where cortisol is secreted) to chill out and relax. When peace and calm are reigning in our lives, like on *The Walton's* (Good night, John Boy), this sort of feedback system works wonderfully. But for those of us living pressure cooker lives and not sleeping adequately for many nights on end, cortisol secretion can quickly get out of control and override this built-in feedback system. As a result, cortisol levels remain elevated around the clock, and can both nag at our blood vessels and nix our weight loss efforts.

Sleep deprivation is an independent risk factor for weight gain. This is because elevated cortisol levels stir the pot of our hunger hormones. Studies have shown that sleep deprivation causes the appetite-controlling hormone, leptin, to fall, and the appetite-stimulating hormone, ghrelin, to increase—the opposite of what we want.[234] It's not surprising then, that when we go without sleep, our appetites can get out of control. Since leptin also regulates our energy expenditure, lower leptin levels following sleep deprivation causes us to conserve energy and fosters fat storage (fig. 9.2). In this way, inadequate sleep not only feels worse than hunger, but it can also actually make us hungry and lead to unwanted weight gain.

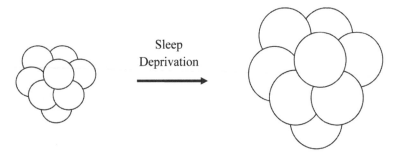

Sleep
Deprivation

Fig. 9.2 Sleep Deprivation Increases Fat Storage

Many medical experts believe that our current obesity epidemic may be in part related to sleep deprivation and the resultant hormonal aberrations that going without shut-eye cause.[235] Their assertion is supported by the dramatic rise in societal obesity over the last number of decades and the parallel trend in shorter sleep duration. Growing laboratory and epidemiological evidence demonstrates that as we've trimmed down our sleep duration, we've added to our waist circumferences.[236] And, the future looks bleak. Never before has this planet seen so many sleep-deprived children, and never before so many that are overweight. Sleep deprivation in childhood has now become a recognized predictor for the development of adult obesity.[237] There's no question that we need to step up our interventions to reduce obesity in children and adults. However, targeting weight management strategies without simultaneously addressing health issues like inadequate sleep is unlikely to prove very effective.

Are You Getting Enough?

Responding to the sentiment that twenty-five years is an impressive duration for a marriage to last, Bob Harris (played by Bill Murray, in Sofia Coppola's *Lost in Translation*) says, "Well, you figure you sleep one-third of your life; that knocks out eight years of marriage right there. So, now you're down to sixteen years and change. You know you're just a teenager at marriage; you can drive it, but there's still the occasional accident." Occasional accidents and marriage aside, it's sobering to think that we sleep away *one-third* of our lives. Considering that our current life expectancy in Canada is about eighty years, that means if we ripen well, we can expect to spend over a quarter of a century sleeping. That's even longer than Rip Van Winkle's epic nap! But sleeping one-third of our lives assumes that we're getting eight hours of sleep every night. Current data suggest this isn't the case. The National Sleep Foundation, for example, revealed that the average adult in the United States sleeps less than seven hours per night, and many far less.[238] Of concern here is the relationship between sleep duration and longevity. As it turns out if one is shortened, so is the other. Epidemiological studies have shown that sleeping less than seven hours per night is associated with a higher mortality rate.[239] While optimal sleep duration may vary somewhat among adults, it's been demonstrated that our brain function is only efficient for about sixteen consecutive hours.[240] Beyond this we can expect to 'zone out' during our activities, and even micro-doze, with repeated brief lapses in alertness. Twenty hours without sleep gets really bad and produces a slowed reaction time, similar to that of an impaired driver. Not surprisingly, the American National Highway Traffic Safety Administration cites sleep deprivation as the cause for over 100,000 crashes, injuries, and fatalities each year.[241] It's one thing to roll over in your sleep while in bed, but quite another while cruising on down the road.

To check and see if you're getting sufficient sleep, take a look at the questionnaire below (table 9.2). For the situations listed, rate your likelihood of falling asleep, between zero, for "never," and three, for "definite." If your answers to the questions tally up to over six, it will be important to give some serious consideration to how you might improve your sleep quantity and quality. If your score is over ten, you've got real trouble and should make an appointment with your family doctor to discuss your sleepiness, ASAP. Who knows, you could be suffering from a treatable sleeping disorder, like obstructive sleep apnea, and not even know it.

Situation	Chance of Sleeping Score 0 = never 1 = slight 2 = moderate 3 = definite
Sitting and reading	
Watching TV	
Sitting inactive in a public place	
Being a passenger in a vehicle for over an hour	
Lying down in the afternoon	
Sitting and talking with someone	
Sitting quietly after lunch (no alcohol)	
Stopped for a few minutes in traffic while driving	
Total score	**Interpretation**
1—6	Rested
7—8	Borderline
9—10	Sleep Deprived
>10	At Risk for Sleep Disorder

Table 9.2 Epworth Sleepiness Score[242]

Suffocating Sleep

Interrupted sleep is a risk factor for both obesity and cardiovascular disease. Sleep-disordered breathing describes a group of disorders characterized by interrupted sleep and includes trouble in the form of breathing pauses or reduced quantity of ventilation during slumber. Sleep-disordered breathing problems are common, affecting approximately one-quarter of Canadian men and nearly 10 percent of women between the ages of thirty and sixty years. One of the more frequent forms of sleep-disordered breathing is called obstructive sleep apnea, estimated to affect one in five North American adults.[243] Obstructive sleep apnea produces symptoms of recurrent morning headaches, daytime fatigue, and failing memory, and often worsens with age; so, if left unattended, obstructive sleep apnea can rob the golden years of their golden slumber.

Obstructive sleep apnea is characterized by the repetitive interruption of respiratory airflow, or ventilation, during sleep. This interruption can be a partial obstruction, like Wheezy the asthmatic squeeze penguin exhibited in *Toy Story*, or a complete obstruction, like former President George W. Bush demonstrated with a pretzel. In either case, the interruption of airflow that occurs in folks with obstructive sleep apnea is due to soft tissue blocking the windpipe. By soft tissue, I'm referring to the tongue, the soft palate, and the uvula (you know, that dangly, reddish thing that hangs down in the back of your throat). Under normal circumstances, the passage of air from the nose and mouth on the outside, to the lungs on the inside, is free and clear of obstruction. However, when the mouth is relaxed during sleep, this oral tissue can potentially collapse in on the windpipe and disrupt airflow. The telltale indicator of partial airway obstruction during sleep is the sound of snoring. While not all snorers have sleep apnea, virtually all patients with obstructive sleep apnea snore. Although obstructive sleep apnea isn't gender-specific and can occur in individuals of every shape and size, it's overweight and middle-aged men who are primarily affected by this condition. This is because men tend to have more generously proportioned oral tissues which can relax and obstruct airflow during sleep.

When the crowded oral tissues relax sufficiently to completely block airflow, breathing comes to an abrupt standstill, producing the sound of silence. But it's not Simon and Garfunkel's "Hello darkness, my old friend" kind of silence. It's a serious suffocating silence that can potentially incite blood vessel injury. The longer this "no airflow" state continues, the more severe the obstruction and the longer the poor spouse is left wondering, "Did you snore off your mortal coil, Honey?" When the breathing pause exceeds ten seconds, medics call it an obstructive apnea ("pnea" means "breath," and "a" refers to "none-at-all").[244] During these apneic episodes, when breathing is obstructed completely, blood oxygen levels drop, and the metabolic waste product, carbon dioxide, builds up. Fortunately for both the sleeper and the worried spouse listening expectantly, breathing generally resumes. This is because the brain is hardwired to detect rising carbon dioxide levels. When carbon dioxide levels reach a certain threshold in the bloodstream, sleep is temporarily interrupted, allowing the obstructed sleeper to rouse enough to take a needed breath. Once oxygen and carbon dioxide levels normalize, sleep resumes—at least until the tongue relaxes again, obstructs airflow, and interrupts sleep once more. Repeated airflow obstructions through the night can lead to severe reductions in blood oxygen levels and marked elevations in carbon dioxide retention. During episodes of apnea, oxygen saturations have been noted to drop by over 60 percent of normal. This low oxygen state, called *hypoxia,* causes the stress hormones, adrenaline and cortisol, to be released into circulation. They in turn cause blood pressure to skyrocket, heart rate to accelerate, and blood vessels to narrow; all of which place considerable strain on our blood vessels when they are supposed to be in a state of rest and repair. This hemodynamic stress can produce electrical instability and accelerate atherosclerosis, either of which can trigger cardiovascular events.[245]

The definitive means to establish the diagnosis of obstructive sleep apnea is best accomplished by way of overnight observation in a laboratory equipped for a formal sleep study. Unfortunately, the diagnosis of obstructive sleep apnea is often delayed. More than 85 percent of patients with clinically significant and treatable obstructive sleep apnea have never been diagnosed.[246] Oftentimes, it's the sleep-deprived, haggard bed partner, with glazed-over eyes who finally brings their hubby's symptoms of suffocating sleep to medical attention. And it's important that someone does because it's potentially lethal. Left untreated, obstructive sleep apnea is associated with a 70 percent increase in the risk of heart disease and stroke (fig. 9.3).[247]

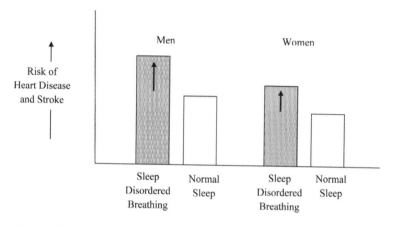

Fig. 9.3 Risk of Vascular Disease with Sleep Disordered Breathing[248]

Too Tired to Sleep

Similar to Robby Burns' dinner grace that "Some hae meat and canna eat, / And some would eat that want it," there are some people who can easily sleep but don't take the time to, while others take the time, but for the life of them, cannot. Those people in the "cannot" group may have the best of intentions, retiring to bed early, donning their comfy flannel jammies, and drawing their blinds tight, but to no avail. They lie in their creaky beds, wide awake into the long and lonely night. It's a horrible feeling, right up there with having a root canal procedure while *Muskrat Love* by Captain and Tennille is playing on the overhead. Over three million Canadians suffer from insomnia and ten times that number in the United States.[249] That's a lot of people left tossing and turning in their beds. As F. Scott Fitzgerald empathized, "The worst thing in the world is to try to sleep and not to." And it's the worst thing for the heart, as well. Studies have shown that people with insomnia are at a higher risk for developing cardiovascular disease and stroke than those who sleep soundly.[250]

Most people suffering from insomnia have difficulty with sleep initiation, which can be related to a variety of things: from racing thoughts about running up your MasterCard to racing thoughts about your teenager running up your MasterCard. By contrast, some people with insomnia are able to fall asleep initially, but then have trouble staying there. It's a no less aggravating form of insomnia, experienced by those with restless legs, overfull bladders, snoring spouses, or a Bavarian cuckoo clock. Sleeping pills may be a useful temporary solution to help bring on sleep, but their long term use can interrupt normal sleep patterns and lead to dependency.

I've had my struggles with insomnia over the years. There were nights, despite feeling dead tired from being on call the night before when I would be unable to fall asleep. Even though I was carrying a large sleep debt and dearly wanted to catch up on my back payments, I would lie there wide awake with my sleep account left in arrears. It might seem like a peculiar problem, being "too tired to sleep," but it was my recurring nightmare, and easily explained. As a result of being overtired, my cortisol stress hormone levels were elevated. So, instead of being able to relax and roll with sleep, I was revved up and ready to rock. It was enough to send me into a panic. "I need to sleep, dammit!" I would cry out in the night. "I'm on call again tomorrow. So, if I don't get some sleep tonight, then when will I!?" I would try to calm myself down and often used a relaxation trick my dad taught me, relaxing each muscle progressively from my toes to my nose. Sometimes, I would resort to taking a hot bath, sipping some lemon tea, reading Dostoyevsky's *The Brothers Karamazov*, and even doing some deep breathing exercises. But, more often than not, nothing seemed to help me sleep. I just couldn't seem to relax enough to pull my attention away from the ticking clock and creaking house to drift off.

In those days, I couldn't afford a string of sleepless nights and was left with little choice but to try a sleeping pill. My family physician, no stranger to the plague of insomnia herself, was empathetic towards my sleep struggles and prescribed me some Lorazepam (Ativan) to "help break a bad cycle." Lorazepam is one of a group of drugs called benzodiazepines ("ben-zoe-dye-as-a-peens"), which affects our brain chemistry enough to induce a state of relaxation— just what I needed. And it seemed to work. I would place the small tablet under my tongue and, within twenty or so minutes, after struggling through another page of Dostoyevsky's dizzying work, I would finally free fall into sleep. So, I took one again the next night, and the next night, and the next. Before I knew it, I *needed* to take an Ativan to sleep. If I didn't have a sleeping pill on board, I wouldn't even consider casting off into sleep. The fleeting thought of not taking a pill would send me into a spin. Holidays were no exception. Even though I was far from the overhead "Stat" pages and frantic pace of the hospital, I needed to taste the powder of that pill under my tongue, or no sandman would even dream of visiting me. I had become, I'm ashamed to say, an Ativan junkie. It wasn't until my stroke, when my injured brain brought with it a crashing wave of fatigue, that I was washed clean of my dependency on sleeping pills and could face the night without any performance-enhancing drugs. So, my advice is to save yourself from the risk of sleeping pill dependency, while there's still time!

Zen and the Art of Sleep/Wake Cycle Maintenance

The popularized Zen saying that "nothing is everything and everything is nothing," might put a spring in one's step while on the road to Nirvana, but on the path to cardiovascular health, it falls short. From the choice and timing of our meals, to the number of steps we walk, and the quantity and quality of our sleep, everything has some effect on our blood vessels, and nothing we do escapes their involvement. When it comes to heart health, a better adage would be "nothing is nothing and everything is something." Since the rhythms of our sleep/wake cycle are intimately tied to our cardiovascular health, we need to do everything in our power to ensure we're getting enough. The following are some practical suggestions that can help to reclaim a frazzled sleep/wake cycle and optimize both cardiovascular health and weight loss efforts. I've divided them into three separate action plans: first, things to put in place before going to bed; second, things to have in place during the night; and third, things to do after awakening to help improve your next night's sleep.

Before Going to Bed

Getting a good night's sleep depends, in part, on what we choose to do during the hour or two before going to bed. We can't rush to sleep, but need to take some time to unwind first, and then slowly ease into slumber. It's like painting your living room. If you want a nice result—smooth and even coverage on the walls, clean-cut lines around the window frames and crown mouldings, and no splatters on the heat registers or green shag carpet—you need to spend some time cleaning the grime off the walls, filling the nail holes in with Polyfilla, and taping around the window sills and trim. Most professional painters insist that the 'prep time' is as important to the final result as rolling on the lavender eggshell itself. So, too, we need to adequately prepare ourselves for our night's rest. To this end, three important points are worth considering.

First, it's important to keep to a regular 'lights out' time. Establishment of a consistent bedtime routine for young children is often recommended to parents, and especially for children with sleep difficulties. But, everyone, young or old, can benefit from a reliable bedtime schedule. If we're always going to bed at a different time of the day and night, a cat nap here, a late night there, our circadian clock receives jumbled messages, confusing our sleep/wake cycle and disrupting our ability to sleep soundly. Just as consistency in business has been recognized as a key quality to long-term financial success; so, too, a consistent bedtime is essential for optimizing our sleep/wake cycle. Hitting the hay at approximately the same time each night (weekends included) reinforces our circadian clock and represents one of the most important sleep hygiene maneuvers.

Second, it's important to avoid any chemicals, drugs, or additives that might interfere with sleep. Nighttime caffeine consumption tops the list. How can we expect to relax and drift off if our hearts are racing to beat the band because of the double shot espresso we had along with that oversized piece of dark chocolate cheesecake after dinner? Forget the cake and, if you must have a coffee, make it a decaf. Caffeine in the form of coffee, tea, chocolate, and colas consumed during the four to six hours before bed is counterproductive to a sound sleep. As well, be aware of the hidden stimulants lurking in the shadows that can steal restorative sleep. For example, many over-the-counter cold remedies contain the stimulant, Synephrine. Such preparations may help keep your nose from dripping, but they're also likely to keep you up. Furthermore, many herbal remedies contain stimulants that can keep you awake... naturally, of course. Examples include Ginseng, Guarana (caffeine), Ma Huang (Ephedra), or Bitter Orange (aka Citrus Aurantium, containing Synephrine). Read the package and choose sleep over substances.

Third, it's important to make every effort to reduce sensory stimulation prior to sleeping. This requires, come evening, that we intentionally protect ourselves from the bombardment of visual and auditory stimulants that bludgeon our senses during the day. We live in a perpetually plugged-in world and all of this late-night Facebook/texting/ Skyping chatter is likely responsible for much of our daytime exhaustion. ("Sup, dude? R U asleep?"). We desperately need to give our henpecking fingers and texting thumbs a rest and turn our electronics to 'sleep' mode so that we can prepare to sleep, as well. That includes turning down the portable music players, like the iPod players, capable of playing music into your ears as loud as Ted Nugent did into mine. Listening to high-intensity noise for long periods can not only result in permanent hearing loss, but it can also impair sleep preparations. Late evening is not the time to start thumbing through your old vinyl collection and playing AC/DC's *Shook me all night long* to shake you all night long. As we settle in for the night, we need to start by dampening the noises of the day, not cranking them up. So, instead of choosing classic rock, go for classic music, instead, and put on Mozart's *Eine Kleine Nacht Musik*, or some of Zamphir's soothing pan flute.

Along the same lines, we're not going to achieve much peace and calm while *Fast and Furious* is blaring on the television set. Late-night television viewing robs us of mental relaxation and sends us further into sleep debt. If you currently have a television set in your bedroom, I strongly suggest moving it somewhere else, like your basement crawl space, or your neighbour's garage sale. Rapid-fire graphic scenes of violence and disturbing storylines counter needed nighttime relaxation. If your hubby wants to watch the evening news and catch the sports highlights from today's big game, just say "Not tonight, Honey, I've got a headache" (Because if anyone like Don Cherry is commentating, you know you're going to have one in short order). Finding out that the Oilers lost to the Leafs four to one, or watching clips of heartbreaking news in the Middle East, isn't going to help your heart any as you try to settle down for sleep. Come morning time, it'll still be "Leafs four, Oilers one," and the world will be as it was, groaning in travail. So, turn down the noise, and turn up the stars.

During the Night

Most adults wake up briefly during the night. This is because we repeatedly cycle through five distinct stages of sleep, each defined by characteristic brainwave activity (table 9.3). It takes about 90 minutes to move from Stage One of drowsy sleep, during which time we're just starting to lose awareness of our surroundings, through to Stage Five, rapid eye movement sleep, or REM, when we have our most vivid dreams.[251] As we make the transit from REM sleep back up to the light sleep of Stage One, and begin a new sleep cycle, our consciousness heightens. During this transient period between sleep cycles, we aren't actually sleeping, and we may become aware of our surroundings.[252] If left undisturbed, we move into another sleep cycle, but if we have a full bladder, a snoring spouse, or a Grandfather clock ticking in the hallway, we may find ourselves fully awake and in that annoying predicament of having to count more sheep.

Sleep Stage	Characteristics	EEG Brain Waveform
Stage 1	Drowsy sleep	Alpha waves
Stage 2	Light sleep	Theta waves
Stage 3	Deep or "slow wave" sleep	Delta waves
Stage 4	Deeper version of Stage 3	Slower Delta waves
Stage 5	Rapid Eye Movement (REM)	Alpha and Beta waves

Table 9.3 Sleep Cycle

To improve my chances of enjoying uninterrupted sleep, I do my utmost to keep things dark, cool and quiet. This means that during the warmer summer months (or a couple of weeks, as is often the case in Edmonton), I open the bedroom window to catch some cooling breeze, don my eyeshades to block out the dawn's early morning rays, and I insert some earplugs to dampen the outdoor noises of late-night traffic and 24-hour road construction. Occasionally, however, despite my best efforts to control my sleeping environment, I resurface to an alert and orientated state well before my intended time to rise and shine. This can be an unnerving time, especially if I have a big day planned. But, as Franklin D. Roosevelt said to an anxious generation, "The only thing we have to fear is fear itself." Understanding how the sleep cycle works has helped diminish my fear of waking up in the night and getting into a tizzy during times of unwanted wakefulness. I've found it quite freeing to know that we don't have to have a completely uninterrupted sleep to reap the benefits of a healthy night's rest. The key factor responsible for making us feel refreshed upon awakening isn't just the length of time asleep, but the number of 90-minute sleep cycles that we complete during the night. Restorative sleep is still possible, even if we briefly awaken between these cycles to stare at the ceiling, so long as we return to sleep in due course and continue on with another cycle. This means, for example, that a person who sleeps for three sleep cycles (roughly 4 ½ hours of sleep), awakens briefly to let in the cat, and then falls asleep again to complete one more cycle (a total of six hours of sleep), will feel more rested than someone with sleep apnea who has been tossing and turning for eight to ten hours in the night, unable to properly complete a single sleep cycle. So, if my peanut-sized bladder happens to stretch enough to waken me in the night, I don't fight it. I calmly shuffle off to the washroom and, once the evacuation is complete, I return to bed, fluff up my pillow, and settle in for 'Round Two' of sleep. If it's half past three in the morning, I know full well that I still have plenty of time for two more complete sleep cycles (roughly 180 minutes) before I need to rise and shine at 7 a.m. Just as General MacArthur kept his promise and returned to his troops, achieving victory in World War II so, too, our slumber will return, if we can relax enough to re-enter Stage One of the next sleep cycle.

"Oh, bullocks!" some chronic insomniacs might counter. "If I wake up in the night, a million ideas come into my head, including how I'm going to be a wreck in the morning if I don't sleep soon. And no matter how hard I try to relax, I know that I'll never fall asleep again!"

True enough; if given a yard, the monkey in our minds can take a mile, and endlessly play with our thoughts throughout the night, whipping them up into concupiscent curds of torment. Griff Niblack joked that "If a man had as many ideas during the day as he does when he has insomnia, he'd make a fortune." So, if I awaken in the night and can't return to sleep within about twenty minutes or so, rather than lying there awake with ideas whirling in my mind a mile a minute, I get out of bed. I find it's better to leave the bedroom and only return once I'm sleepy again. Sleepiness usually returns after I've had a glass of milk or a small bowl of cereal, and

I catch up on some of the latest scientific breakthroughs, in *Scientific American* or my wife's copy of *O, the Oprah Magazine*. I also find that making a brief entry into my journal during those wee hours provides an opportunity to lay down whatever concerns I might have and helps me calm my thoughts for the remainder of the night. Making a list of my worries diffuses their power and gives me the peace of mind to welcome peace into my mind. Upon my return to bed, if sleep still plays hard to get, I settle into the bed nonetheless, comforted by the sure knowledge that although sleeping is better than lying awake; lying awake and calmly resting is still better than having a hissy fit, anxious and frustrated. Relaxation techniques like biofeedback, mental imagery, hypnosis, meditation, and prayer can help improve the chance that slumber will return. But sleep or no sleep, times of relaxation—even if they occur in the middle of the night when you'd rather be catching some shuteye—have important health benefits. Relaxation, in and of itself, can slow heart rates, reduce blood pressure, normalize cortisol levels, and improve vascular function.[253]

After Awaking in the Morning

To optimize our circadian rhythm, consistency is crucial. That means that it's important to keep to a regular wake time in the morning, no matter how short or long we may have slept. So, when the radio alarm clock suddenly blares out Sonny and Cher in the morning ("Babe," *ba-ba ba-ba ba-ba ba* "I got you, Babe," *ba-ba ba-ba ba-ba ba* "I got you, Babe..."), we must avoid burying ourselves under the pillow and hiding, regardless of our current affection for that melody. There's no benefit in procrastinating. Morning is as inevitable as death and inheritance taxes; so, it's best to just get up and face the music, focusing our attention on breaking our fast, rather than breaking our alarm clock.

If you find that your sleep isn't very refreshing, there's no advantage to wallowing in sleep-deprived pity. Instead, give some consideration to how you might improve your sleep quality in the future, namely tonight. Yesterday may be history and tomorrow but a mystery, but tonight could be the night you sleep like a baby and awaken refreshed. Exercise incorporated into your day—today—will be of immense help in making this dream a reality. While strenuous exercise within the two hours before bedtime might rev up your engine a little too much and interfere with your ability to settle down at night, exercise during the daytime is an excellent way to improve sleep. Regular exercise reduces cortisol levels and acts as an important Zeitgeber in the maintenance of an optimal sleep/wake cycle. There's nothing like mildly sore muscles and physical fatigue to make that mattress feel like heaven while rolling out the red carpet for the Sandman.

Marion's Dream Hygiene

"Truth be told," Marion confessed, "I have difficulty getting to sleep, even when Bill uses his CPAP machine and doesn't snore at all."

"I guess the humming of the machine isn't all that lulling," I said.

"No, the noise of the CPAP machine doesn't bother me," she countered. "I just have difficulty relaxing. So, I usually take a Zopiclone (Immovane). I just know I won't sleep otherwise, so I take a pill right away, often while the late-night news is still on."

"Interestingly, sometimes sleeping pills can actually cause agitation and even nightmares," I informed Marion. "But, your difficulty relaxing at night probably has more to do with your bedtime routine, including watching television."

"Television is something my husband and I can do together," she said in defense.

"I'm sure the two of you can think of better things to do together," I said with a grin. "And besides, studies have shown that the two key culprits for sleep deprivation in our society are late-night television viewing and early morning work schedules.[254] Now, not everyone can modify their morning start times at work, but there should be no excuses for curbing late-night television."

"Well, as a global citizen, I think that watching the world news and keeping informed are essential," Marion retorted.

"Maybe so, but proper sleep is also essential," I countered. "Sleep is when your blood vessels get repaired and when your weight loss efforts can be enhanced. So, it's important to do everything possible to ensure you're getting all forty of your winks."

"Television or no television," Marion said, shaking her head. "I don't think that I'll be able to sleep without taking a pill to relax, first."

"You don't have to go cold turkey on your sleeping pills," I reassured her. "But, in the long run, sleeping aids can interfere with our natural sleep/wake cycle by not allowing us to properly cycle through all five stages of sleep, and can be counterproductive to restorative sleep; so, I'd avoid them if possible. Why don't you start by tapering the dose, like taking half a pill tonight? You could also consider switching to a milder sedative, like Nytol's valerian root, as a transition medication. And some attention to sleep hygiene can also help re-establish your sleep/wake cycle," I said, as I handed her a copy of Table 9.4, below. "If you really must have some evening entertainment, turn off the computer and television and try an audiobook. And, instead of world news, choose something on the lighter side. A good belly laugh and a proper sleep are a couple of my favorite means to optimize health."

Regular bedtime	Retire at a similar time each evening, including weekends
	Avoid long naps during the day (> 30 min)
	Avoid late nights
Environment	Use darkening blinds or eye shields
	Keep the room cool and well ventilated
	Keep the room quiet with earplugs, white noise machine, turning phone volume down
	Use the bedroom for only sleep and sex, not work or television
	Practice relaxation techniques like deep breathing
No sensory stimulation	Read or journal instead of screen time
	Turn down the music
	Turn off the computer and TV
Eliminate chemicals	Alcohol impairs the normal sleep cycle
	Caffeine, especially during the 4-6 hours before bed (Coffee, tea, colas, chocolate, and some herbals)
	Synephrine (cold remedies and some herbals)
	Sleeping pills
Wake time	Plan to rise at a similar time every day (including weekends)
	Avoid having to use an alarm clock
	Get up as soon as you wake up

Table 9.4 RENEW Sleep Hygiene Tips

Chapter Summary
The Beauty of Rest

- A healthy sleep pattern constitutes a series of sleep cycles, each lasting approximately 90 minutes

- A sleep cycle is made up of five distinct sleep stages (drowsiness through to rapid eye movement or REM sleep) each defined by characteristic brainwave activity

- Sleep aids can interfere with our natural sleep/wake cycle and cause unrefreshed sleep by preventing the repeated cycling of all five stages of sleep

- The Epworth Sleepiness Score can help identify those with an inadequate sleep pattern

- Symptoms of ADHD are related to excessive television and computer use and associated with difficulty in controlling weight

- The Adult Attention-Deficit/Hyperactivity Disorder (ADHD) Self-reporting

- CPAP for patients with obstructive sleep apnea improves metabolic health and helps weight loss

- The bedroom should be reserved for sex and sleep only (no computer or television!)

- To assist returning to sleep in the middle of the night, don't attempt to force sleep, but get out of bed immediately and engage the mind and tire the eyes by reading

- On return to bed, discipline your mind to focus only on what was read, and not to wander or think about the worries of the day ahead
- RENEW Sleep Hygiene Tips—Regular bedtime, Environmental optimization, No television before bed, Elimination of chemicals, and Waking up at a regular time—can help restore a healthy sleep pattern

Chapter Notes

222. Cortese S, Angriman M, Maffeis C, Isnard P, Konofal E, Lecendreux M, Purper-Ouakil D, Vincenzi B, Bernardina BD, Mouren MC. Attention-deficit/hyperactivity disorder (ADHD) and obesity: a systematic review of the literature. Crit Rev Food Sci Nutr. 2008 Jun;48(6):524-37.

223. Wender PH. Attention-deficit/hyperactivity disorder in adults. Psychiatric Clinics of North America. 1998;21:761-774.

224. Pagoto SL, Curtin C, Lemon SC, Bandini LG, Schneider KL, Bodenlos JS, Ma Y. Association between adult attention deficit/hyperactivity disorder and obesity in the US population. Obesity (Silver Spring). 2009 Mar;17(3):539-44.

225. Kessler RC, Adler LA, Gruber MJ, Sarawate CA, Spencer T, Van Brunt DL. Validity of the World Health Organization Adult ADHD Self-Report Scale (ASRS) Screener in a representative sample of health plan members. Int J Methods Psychiatr Res. 2007;16(2):52-65.

226. Kessler RC, Adler L, Ames M, Demler O, Faraone S, Hiripi E, Howes MJ, Jin R, Secnik K, Spencer T, Ustun TB, Walters EE. The World Health Organization Adult ADHD Self-Report

Scale (ASRS): a short screening scale for use in the general population. Psychol Med. 2005 Feb;35(2):245-56.

227. Tao ZL, Liu Y. Is there a relationship between Internet dependence and eating disorders? A comparison study of Internet dependents and non-Internet dependents. Eat Weight Disord. 2009 Jun-Sep;14(2-3):e77-83.

228. Cortese S, Konofal E, Dalla Bernardina B, Mouren MC, Lecendreux M. Does excessive daytime sleepiness contribute to explaining the association between obesity and ADHD symptoms? Med Hypotheses. 2008;70(1):12-6.

229. Martin JM, Carrizo SJ, Vicente E, Agusti AG. Long term cardiovascular outcomes in men with obstructive sleep apnoea-hypopnoea with or without treatment with continuous positive airway pressure: an observational study. Lancet. 2005;365:1046-1053.

230. Loube DI, Loube AA, Erman MK. Continuous positive airway pressure treatment results in weight loss in overweight and obese patients with obstructive sleep apnea. J of Am Diet Assoc 1997;97(8):896-897.

231. Menachem Begin. White nights: The story of a prisoner in Russia. Harper 1979.

232. Atkeson A, Yeh SY, Malhotra A, Jelic S. Endothelial function in obstructive sleep apnea. Prog Cardiovasc Dis. 2009 Mar-Apr;51(5):351-62.

233. William Shakespeare Macbeth Scene 2, Act 2, Lines 36-39.

234. Spiegel K, Tasali E, Penev P, Van Cauter E. Brief communication: Sleep curtailment in healthy young men is associated with decreased leptin levels, elevated ghrelin levels, and increased hunger and appetite. Ann Intern Med. 2004 Dec 7;141(11):846-50.

235. Chen X, Beydoun MA, Wang Y. Is sleep duration associated with childhood obesity? A systematic review and meta-

analysis. Obesity (Silver Spring). 2008 Feb;16(2):265-74.

236. Van Cauter E, Knutson KL. Sleep and the epidemic of obesity in children and adults. Eur J Endocrinol. 2008 Dec;159 Suppl 1:S59-66.

237. Gangwisch JE, Malaspina D, Boden-Albala B, Heymsfield SB. Inadequate sleep as a risk factor for obesity: analyses of the NHANES I. Sleep. 2005 Oct 1;28(10):1289-96.

238. National Sleep Foundation. 2005. Sleep in America Poll: summary of findings. Available from http://www.sleepfoundation.org/content/hottopics/2005.

239. Kripke DF, Garfinkel L, Wingard DL, Klauber MR, Marler MR. Mortality associated with sleep duration and insomnia. Arch Gen Psychiatry 2002;59:131-136.

240. Iglowstein I, Jenni OG, Molinari L, Largo RH. Sleep duration from infancy to adolescence: reference values and generational trends. Pediatrics. 2003 Feb;111(2):302-7.

241. Vaca F. National Highway Traffic Safety Administration (NHTSA) notes. Drowsy driving. Ann Emerg Med. 2005 Apr;45(4):433-4.

242. Johns MW. A new method for measuring daytime sleepiness: the Epworth sleepiness scale. Sleep 1991. 14 (6): 540–5.

243. Young T, Peppard PE, Gottlieb DJ. Epidemiology of obstructive sleep apnea: a population health perspective. Am J Respir Crit Care Med. 2002;165:1217-1239.

244. Sleep-related breathing disorders in adults: recommendations for syndrome definition and measurement techniques in clinical research. The Report of an American Academy of Sleep Medicine Task Force. Sleep. 1999;22:667-689.

245. Somers VK, Dyken ME, Clary MP, Abboud FM. Sympathetic neural mechanisms in obstructive sleep apnea. J Clin Invest. 1995;96:1897-1904.

246. Kapur v, Strohl KP, Redline S, Iber C, O'Connor G, Neito J. Under-diagnosis of sleep apnea syndrome in U.S. communities. Sleep Breath. 2002;6:49-54.

247. Marin JM, Carrizo SJ, Vicente E, Agusti AG. Long-term cardiovascular outcomes in men with obstructive sleep apnoea-hypopnoea with or without treatment with continuous positive airway pressure: an observational study. Lancet, 2005;365: 1046-53.

248. Mooe T, Franklin KA, Holmstrom K, Rabben T, Wiklund. Sleep-disordered breathing and coronary artery disease: long term prognosis. Am J Respir Crit Care Med 2001;164:1910-1913.

249. Ting L, Malhotra A. Disorders of sleep: an overview. Prim Care. 2005 Jun;32(2):305-18, v.

250. Mindell JA, Meltzer LJ, Carskadon MA, Chervin RD. Developmental aspects of sleep hygiene: findings from the 2004 National Sleep Foundation Sleep in America Poll. Sleep Med. 2009 Aug;10(7):771-9.

251. Murillo-Rodríguez E, Arias-Carrión O, Sanguino-Rodríguez K, González-Arias M, Haro R. Mechanisms of sleep-wake cycle modulation. CNS Neurol Disord Drug Targets. 2009 Aug;8(4):245-53.

252. Merica H, Fortune RD. State transitions between wake and sleep, and within the ultradian cycle, with focus on the link to neuronal activity. Sleep Med Rev. 2004 Dec;8(6):473-85.

253. Bernardi L, Sleight P, Bandinelli G, Cencetti S, Fattorini L, Wdowczyc-Szulc J, Lagi A. Effect of rosary prayer and yoga mantras on autonomic cardiovascular rhythms: comparative study. BMJ 2001;323:1446-1449.

254. Basner M, Dinges DF. Dubious bargain: trading sleep for Leno and Letterman. Sleep. 2009 Jun 1;32(6):747-52.

Chapter 10
Weight Control Fast
Utility and Practice of Intermittent Fasting

When Less is More

I glanced over my afternoon clinic schedule and saw Marion's name at the top of the list. It had been some time since I last saw her, so, to refresh my memory, I read over my last consult letter. "Hmmm… I wonder how she's made out with those risk factors and her weight control?" I asked myself, as I donned my stethoscope and knocked on the door.

"Long time no see," I said with a smile, as I entered the consultation room. She was seated on the examination table with the blood pressure cuff secured to her arm.

"That's the last reading now," she replied, nodding to the automated BP monitor, as it completed the final measurement. "The first one was quite a bit higher, but this is more like what I get at home."

"Glad to hear it," I said. "The first reading is often an outlier—all that rushing about to get here. But, 124/84 mmHg is an excellent blood pressure measurement. You must be doing some things right, eh, with your meds and low-salt diet?"

"Yes, my blood pressure's been pretty good since the last medication adjustment. That's not the problem; it's my cholesterol and sugar control... not to mention my weight," she said with a tone of frustration. "I've seen a dietician as you suggested, and my husband and I have been trying to follow her advice. We gave up fast food and even took out gym memberships. But, I've still got a long way to go to start getting rid of all this," she added, motioning to her abdomen and thighs.

"Good for you," I said with encouragement. "Those are some really important steps that you've made, and together no less."

"Yes, I figured you'd like hearing that. We've both lost some weight. Cutting out the late-night snacking was probably most helpful for me, but I'm still a long way from a healthy weight. Isn't there anything else I can do?"

"I suppose, but sometimes less is more," I responded. "Rather than doing more to improve your weight control, maybe it's time to do less. If you've got your dietary ducks in a row, and a regular exercise regimen in place, perhaps some intermittent fasting is in order."

"Fasting?!" Marion exclaimed. "I thought fasting was bad for you... lowers your metabolic rate and causes you to lose water and muscle..."

"Yes, you're right," I affirmed. "Prolonged fasting can have adverse effects on the body. Mahatma Gandhi fasted for political reasons not personal health. But. *intermittent* fasting is a different matter. Two or three 16-hour fasts in the week can greatly improve your weight control and even bring your cholesterol and blood sugar levels into line. Mind you, only if a prudent diet is followed and resistance exercises are undertaken regularly. Otherwise, any benefits gained are for not."

Extending the Benefits of Rest

The mechanism for how intermittent fasting benefits our health includes its influence on our circadian rhythm. The circadian rhythm regulates hormones, physiologic processes, and coordinates metabolism, as well as our energy utilization.[255] During periods of wakefulness and food consumption, there is a release of the anabolic hormones, insulin and ghrelin. Insulin regulates our blood sugar levels by assisting the entrance of glucose into our cells, and ghrelin, our hunger hormone, stimulates appetite. Both insulin and ghrelin promote fat storage, particularly abdominal fat—not something we desire. Conversely, when we are sleeping or are in a fasted state, insulin and ghrelin levels drop off. During these times of snoozing and fasting, there is a release of glucagon and leptin, instead. By contrast to insulin and ghrelin, which promote pudge procurement, glucagon and leptin free up fat for burning. These catabolic hormones have the opposite effect on our energy stores, breaking down and mobilizing fat, and making it available as a fuel source for energy production. Optimal health and weight control necessitate the care and maintenance of these natural rhythms and hormonal processes.

One of the major contributors to our obesity epidemic in North America is the disruption of our circadian rhythm.[256] As discussed in the last chapter, inadequate sleep can throw off our natural biological clock, causing our hunger hormone to rise, satiety hormone to fall and, among other troubles, lead to weight gain. But, sleep disturbance isn't the only way our clock gets a knock. The timing of our meals also affects our circadian rhythm, especially if our meals are occurring all the time. This is because food acts as a powerful *Zietgeber*— an external time cue for our circadian rhythm. Similar to light exposure, physical activity, ambient temperature, and noise, food consumption provides important feedback to the master clock of our brains, which adjusts our circadian rhythm accordingly, effecting the biological synchrony of our energy balance. With the rise of convenience foods and the dismantling of the family dinner hour, there has been a general blurring of the borders separating mealtimes. Eating between meals has become normalized in our culture— eating at work, eating at play, eating at the computer, eating at the park, eating in transit, eating, eating, and more eating. It's like a 24/7 graze craze. As a result, we're not only living under extended periods of wakefulness, we're living under extended periods of ingestion events, too. Similar to how difficult it is to sleep when it's always daytime, like at the Arctic Circle during the spring equinox, for example, stretching out caloric consumption throughout the day confuses our biological clock. Grazing behavior not only inundates our bodies with unnecessary calories (many of which are of low quality or even empty calories), it disrupts our circadian rhythm and sets the stage for cardiovascular disease and weight gain.

This is where intermittent fasting comes to the rescue. In addition to what we can do to optimize sleep hygiene and reign in our grazing behaviour, intermittent fasting can be helpful in re-establishing our circadian rhythm and setting us back on a path towards metabolic health and weight control. It does so by two means. First, intermittent fasting effectively extends our nocturnal hormonal milieu into our waking and working hours. By remaining in an entirely fasted state, we can keep our insulin and ghrelin levels on the low and napping. All the while, our catabolic hormones, glucagon and leptin—which will continue to be released and active in our circulation if we eat nothing—can get at our fat stores and mobilize them for energy. The key is to consume absolutely zero calories—not even artificial sweeteners that mimic sugar and fool our senses into awakening insulin release. This way, so long as we remain fasting, fat gets burned.

Secondly, intermittent fasting helps to reset our biological clock. Providing a time-restricted window for eating imposes a diurnal rhythm for food intake, resulting in improved oscillations of our circadian clock. Like having distinct nighttimes and daytimes improves our sleep cycle, this sharp demarcation between eating and not eating sends clear messages to the master clock of our brains, allowing for appropriate adjustments to meet our metabolic demands. Analogous to correcting your wristwatch using the time on your cellphone, these feasting/fasting adjustments function to reset our biological clocks, leading to optimized metabolic function. It's a timely rescue. This resynchronization of the circadian rhythm is increasingly being recognized as an important avenue for the prevention of cardiovascular disease and obesity.[257]

Two-Compartment Model

We have two main energy compartments in our body: glycogen, located primarily in our liver and muscle cells; and body fat, located around our abdominal organs and viscera, and ... well... in places where we don't particularly want fat to be located, like the hips, thighs, backside... you get the picture. Our body makes use of these energy stores to provide needed fuel for our metabolic needs and activities of the day. While both compartments are accessible, the body tends to prefer using our glycogen stores for day-to-day function, and keep the fat stores as a backup, in case of a famine in the land. The reason for this favoritism because fat is stored storage in expensive real estate. Fat storage is extremely energy efficient and requires remarkably little space. Unlike glycogen which needs to be stored alongside a significant proportion of bulky water, fatty acids can line up snug and streamlined, no water needed. And, unlike glycogen—our high-maintenance, quick and clean fuel—fat storage is a rather underwhelming, low-energy affair. By comparison to glycogen, fat cells are relatively docile and metabolically inactive—you just feed 'em and forget 'em. So, depending on our caloric intake and activity level, we tend to turn over our glycogen stores regularly, and progressively pack away the pounds in the form of body fat.

In his book, *The Complete Guide to Fasting*, Dr. Jason Fung, a Canadian nephrologist with interest in nutrition, likens these two energy compartments to that of a fridge and a freezer.[258] The glycogen storehouse is compared to a fridge, in that it's not too big, easy to access, and useful for moment-to-moment needs, like grabbing a quick bite or getting a glass of orange juice. By comparison, our fat storehouse is compared to a freezer. This is because a freezer is large enough for ample cold storage but is typically located downstairs in the unfinished basement, and is a bit of an inconvenience to access. So, the trick with any weight reduction method is to encourage our body to go downstairs to the freezer and access our fat stores for energy, rather than just grabbing some quick glycogen from the fridge. Attention to prudent diet and adoption of an exercise regimen can do this to a certain degree. However, as experienced dieters will attest, weight loss achievements by lifestyle changes are hard-won. Fortunately, intermittent fasting performs this very efficiently and ideally complements our prudent lifestyle choices. Although there's no sleight of hand or black magic involved, the fat-reducing results of intermittent fasting can certainly appear to be magical.

Having a restricted eating window forces fat metabolism. Since the body preferentially uses glycogen as an energy store—a process known as glycogenolysis—it typically takes several hours before body fat begins to get broken down. Once the glycogen stores have been depleted, the body has no choice but to go downstairs to the fat stores in the freezer for energy. After approximately 12 hours of fasting, the breakdown of fat (called *lipolysis, lipo* for fat and *lysis* for breakdown) shifts into high gear. This transition from using glycogen as the primary energy source to using fat is called *intermittent metabolic switching* (IMS) or glucose-ketone (G-to-K) switchover.[259] This switchover from the use of glucose as the primary fuel source to the use of fatty acids and ketone bodies is more energy efficient for the body and allows for greater metabolic flexibility.[260] In keeping with the adage, *practice makes perfect*, this switchover improves in efficiency with time, occurring earlier in the fast and more smoothly. With body fat bitten, fatty acids and ketones get liberated into the bloodstream and become the main source of energy for cells. The ketone bodies, with their characteristic musty apple odor, account for that less-than-pleasant morning breath on awakening and provide one more reason to brush our pearly whites. The brain, which has the highest metabolic demands of the body, can efficiently utilize ketones for energy without missing a step. In fact, those of us who practice time-restricted fasting concur with the findings that mental clarity, memory, and learning capacity improve with intermittent fasting.[261]

Fasting & Insulin Sensitivity

One of the most important health benefits of time-restricted eating is the effect it has on insulin sensitivity. As mentioned in Chapter 4, *Enlisting Lunch*, diabetes represents a serious risk factor for the development of cardiovascular disease and stroke, and is increasing in prevalence in our society. So, prevention is key. Type 2 diabetes, which is the most common form of diabetes, is caused by progressive insulin resistance—the body develops a tolerance to insulin and doesn't respond to it as needed. By contrast to type 1 diabetes, which is marked by immune-mediated pancreatic injury causing insulin deficiency, in type 2 diabetes the pancreas produces adequate amounts of insulin, but without effect. The insulin receptors lose their sensitivity to insulin, and as a result, are unable to effectively bind the hormone, so it can do its job, transporting glucose into cells. Like a celebrity making an appearance at a natural disaster scene, insulin is present but not particularly useful or effective. As a result, blood glucose levels rise and, over time, cause vascular damage, and can lead to heart disease and stroke.

Ironically, the common remedy of using insulin to treat type 2 diabetes completely misses the mark and is even counterproductive. The problem in type 2 diabetes is not a lack of insulin; it's a lack of insulin effect. So, what's fundamentally needed isn't more insulin, but an improvement in insulin sensitivity. Although there are medications now available that can address this, they don't get to the root of the problem. Why is there insulin resistance in the first place? In brief, it's because of the increased amounts of abdominal fat. Our visceral fat stores, as mentioned in Chapter 3, Coffee Break Caution, produce inflammatory mediators that counter the effects of insulin. So, what's needed isn't more insulin and an increase in medications, but fewer calories and decreased abdominal fat. Lifestyle measures, in the form of weight-reducing diet and regular exercise, get to the root issue and are proven effective in significantly countering insulin resistance. Unfortunately, following a prudent diet and exercise regimen can be challenging for most, with slow improvements hard gained. As a result, the problem of insulin resistance often persists and, in time, can worsen.

Intermittent fasting might be just the answer to both address the root issue and allow for regaining insulin sensitivity. Observational population studies have shown cardiovascular and metabolic benefits of intermittent fasting, with improvements in the handling of insulin and glucose.[262] Studies have even shown that time-restricted fasting improves receptor sensitivity to insulin and occurs independently of weight loss.[263] This improvement in insulin sensitivity relates to the reduced insulin levels that result from the fasted state. When insulin levels are kept low, receptors to the hormone can recover and become revitalized. In time, the body can regain its sensitivity to insulin and end the downward spiral of hyperglycemia. With diminished insulin resistance comes normalized blood glucose levels and a reduction in vascular injury. It's a win-win scenario: improved weight control and improved glycemic control. Knowing this, intermittent fasting should be seen as an effective complement to the proven beneficial effects of lifestyle maneuvers on countering insulin resistance.

Metabolic Health & More

The health benefits of intermittent fasting go beyond weight control and even the improvement in insulin sensitivity and include demonstrable improvements in numerous metabolic parameters, endothelial vascular function, and gastrointestinal wellbeing. To help bring these various benefits to mind during my discussions with patients, I make use of the acronym, FASTING, as outlined below (Table 10.1).

F	Fat burning
A	Anti-inflammatory effect
S	Synchronization of circadian rhythm
T	Total cholesterol reduction
I	Insulin sensitivity
N	Normalization of blood pressure
G	Gastrointestinal health

Table 10.1 Benefits of Intermittent Fasting

As outlined in Chapter 6, *In Defense of Afternoon Snacking*, the endothelial cells that line the inside surface of our blood vessels play an integral role in maintaining vascular health. Our diet and activity level can greatly affect these cells, both positively and negatively. In addition to choosing fresh fruits and vegetables for snacking options, for example, intermittent fasting has been shown to significantly enhance endothelial function. Numerous mechanisms are considered to be responsible for this improvement in vascular function. Part of this is thought to be related to the weight loss that occurs with intermittent fasting; part is due to the reduced production of damaging free radicals and resultant oxidation; and, part is secondary to the anti-inflammatory effects of intermittent fasting.[264] These broad and beneficial actions occur because ketone bodies aren't just fasting fuel; they are potent signaling molecules that have major effects on cellular and organ function, including countering the effects of oxidation and inflammation.[265] In addition, intermittent fasting has shown significant modulating effects on well-defined cardiovascular risk factors. Studies have shown that patients who follow a time-restricted fasting protocol have significant reductions in triglyceride values, as well as levels of LDL cholesterol (bad cholesterol).[266] This discovery has opened up a novel lifestyle approach for augmenting the treatment of elevated cholesterol levels. What's more, blood pressure control has also been shown to improve in patients who follow a time-restricted eating/fasting dietary regimen. Like regular exercise, intermittent fasting acts as a panacea for cardiometabolic health.

In addition to the cardiovascular benefits of intermittent

fasting, this dietary approach has been shown to improve gastrointestinal health, as well. Our intestinal health depends, to a great extent, on the groups of microorganisms, or microbiota, that live there—fermenting fiber, synthesizing essential amino acids and vitamins, and maintaining normal function, referred to as gut homeostasis.[267] Numerous disease states, including the metabolic syndrome, as discussed in Chapter 3, *Coffee Break Caution*, can damage our gut microbiota, and produce trouble referred to as dysbiosis (*dys* for damaged, and *biosis* for mode of life). Studies have shown that intermittent fasting can shape our intestinal flora, and can not only promote gut health but restore a healthy microbiota.[268] I discovered this myself some years ago after a bout of gastroenteritis. I had made the mistake of eating some raw seafood at a New Year's Eve party and spent the first six months of the year suffering from abdominal cramps and watery diarrhea. After being diagnosed with irritable bowel syndrome, I was instructed to use a combination of Pepto-Bismol and Loperamide, as needed for symptom control. Although the combination of medicines was somewhat helpful, my symptoms completely disappeared after I began to incorporate intermittent fasting into my week. Now, if cramps and diarrhea recur, I snap into action and plan a fast.

Frequent Fasting FAQs

Since our culture is immersed in a graze-craze mindset, the notion of fasting for many of my patients seems to run against the grain. As a result, I occasionally get some push back when I raise the topic and mention the benefits of intermittent fasting. The following are some frequently asked questions that I'm asked in clinic, which are important to address.

Doesn't intermittent fasting reduce the metabolic rate, like starvation?

The sum of physical and chemical processes enlisted to maintain the vital functions of our bodies at rest—you know, respiration, perspiration, and consternation—is called our resting metabolism. If we subtract the activities of food consumption—including slurping, chewing, burping, digestion, and absorption—then we arrive at what's termed our basal metabolism. The rate at which our body tissues metabolize fuel nutrients for energy during these moments of repose (eating and digestion excluded) is referred to as our basal metabolic rate or BMR. Our basal metabolic rates aren't all the same but are individually programmed. Some people, typically the young, buff, athletic types, burn calories faster than older, more sedentary folk. While normal BMR levels for women range between 1100 to 1500 kilocalories per day and 1600 to 1900 kilocalories per day for men, the values can fluctuate significantly, depending on our caloric consumption. When food intake is reduced, our BMR rate follows suit and slows down, producing what's termed the *starvation mode* if the caloric reduction is significant. However, intermittent fasting should not be confused with reduced caloric intake. When we consume zero calories—nil, zip, nada—we turn on our flight-or-fight response, causing the catecholamine stress hormone, norepinephrine, to be released into circulation. This hormone facilitates fat breakdown and the switch from glucose to ketones for fuel. Studies have shown that the BMR and resting energy expenditures actually increase during intermittent fasting.[269] So, if anything, intermittent fasting revs up our metabolism rather than slows it down. This catecholamine release provides an energy boost, as well. Truth be told, this is the real reason that I continue to do intermittent fasting. Even though I achieved an ideal bodyweight years ago, I still plan occasional 16-hour fasts in my week (usually my busiest days) and do so primarily for the energy boost. When I fast, I feel switched on, efficient, clear-headed, and ready for anything.

Isn't there a risk that intermittent fasting can lower blood sugar and cause hypoglycemia?

Although concerns have been raised that intermittent fasting can reduce blood glucose levels into the danger zone—a serious condition known as hypoglycemia—this is really only an issue for those on blood sugar lowering medications. To avoid this, I recommend that my patients with diabetes involve their primary care physician before embarking on a fasting protocol. Frequent monitoring of blood sugar levels is essential—two to four times per day if need be. When done under the supervision of the patient's healthcare professional, and with appropriate glucose monitoring, intermittent fasting can be safely undertaken in patients with diabetes.[270] Generally, blood sugar lowering medicines will need to be held during fasting days, and blood sugar levels allowed to ride a bit higher than usual (optimal blood sugar range 8 to 10 mmol/L on fasting days). Higher levels of blood sugar are far less a problem in the short term than full-blown hypoglycemia, which in severe cases can prove fatal. For those of us not on blood sugar lowering medications, however, the fasted state doesn't case worrisome reductions in blood sugar. The reason being that we don't actually need to eat sugar for our blood sugar levels to remain normal. Our bodies are capable of synthesizing glucose on their own without the need of ingesting a single thing—a process called gluconeogenesis (*neo* for newly and *genesis* to make). Gluconeogenesis keeps blood glucose levels nicely within the normal range during periods of fasting.

Doesn't intermittent fasting burn muscle?

One common concern about fasting is losing muscle. This concern is based on the fact that our bodies make use of amino acids—the protein building blocks—as raw materials for the synthesis of glucose during times of fasting. Our muscle tissue is a major storehouse for cellular protein and amino acids. So, the concern is that in order to synthesize the needed glucose while fasting, the body would be forced to dismantle our all-important muscle tissue. However, dismantling muscles isn't the only source of amino acids. As part of normal cellular function, there is a continual recycling of proteins that occurs in our bodies every day. While some proteins get assembled, others get disassembled. It's nature's way. This recycling process liberates amino acids into circulation and allows for protein conservation to take effect, preserving our lean body mass in general, and muscle tissue, in particular. Studies of patients following alternate-day fasting protocols showed this to be the case. Even after 70 days of fasting one day and feeding the next, participants in the study had no loss of fat-free mass.[271] Nonetheless, loss of muscle can occur if muscles aren't being used. It's the old adage, the *use it or lose it* phenomenon. After 30 years of age, all of us can expect to experience some slow and steady loss of muscle tissue with each passing decade, particularly if we don't exercise. Since this process could possibly be accelerated by following a fasting dietary protocol, it's imperative to have a regular resistance exercise regimen in place before embarking on a fasting schedule. You do not want to lose muscle! It's prime real estate that you earned and need to keep. The health benefits of weight loss are reduced if a portion of the weight that's been lost turns out to be muscle tissue. To prevent muscle loss, I intentionally plan a resistance exercise routine on the morning of my fasting days. Exercising on fasting days is helpful for several reasons. First, it causes our glycogen stores to get consumed faster, and fast tracks fat breakdown. Second, it preserves my lean body mass. By giving my bicep muscles a dose of exercise, for example, I'm telling my body that I need those pipes, and to build them up, rather than tear them down. By exercising regularly—resistance and aerobic training—I have been able to improve my fitness level and build muscle, even though I do intermittent fasting, and even though I'm in the *Silver Senior* age category.

Isn't intermittent fasting problematic because it doesn't teach healthy eating and even promotes overeating?

Intermittent fasting is an advanced dietary strategy. To build health and optimize fat loss, a prudent and portioned diet, as well as a regular exercise regimen need to be in place before incorporating a fasting schedule into one's routine. Intermittent fasting is dependent upon these lifestyle pillars. Any fasting protocol that doesn't pay heed to them is doomed to failure. Weight might be lost, sure, but unless resistance exercise is being done, say good-bye to your muscle mass. And, if a period of fasting is followed by an unbridled junk food fest, then say good-bye, as well, to any metabolic health gains. All efforts will be for not. Inactivity and inept eating undo any fasting headway. So, the problems are with our lifestyle choices, not so much the fasting regimen.

In terms of what intermittent fasting *can* teach us, there is an important lesson, namely the size of the stomach. After 16 hours of fasting, the size of our stomach shrinks considerably. This is due to the lack of incoming food to stretch the stomach, as well as the fasting hormonal milieu, which causes it to contract. So, on breaking such a fast, it doesn't take very much food to feel full. And, it doesn't take very much more food to feel tired. It's like having a sudden post-Thanksgiving feast fatigue. All the vim and vigor enjoyed during the fasting window vanishes, and our get-up-and-go gets up and goes. So, to avoid this, I break my fast with a small bowl of bone broth. It's warm and satisfying, easily absorbed, and gently fills the stomach without causing much stretch. Then, 15 to 20 minutes later, I follow this with a keto-friendly mini-meal, an hour or so before my regular dinner meal. The improved awareness of my stomach size has helped me to better gauge my portion sizes on my non-fasting days, as well.

Doesn't intermittent fasting deprive our bodies of important nutrients?

Fortunately, micronutrient deficiency is rare in developed countries. With the exceptions of childhood, in pregnancy, and while breastfeeding, during which times fasting should be prohibited, intermittent fasting won't interfere with our essential nutrient requirements. Following a time-restricted protocol partitions nutrients, but doesn't eliminate them. There are essential nutrients we need, to be sure, which include vitamins, minerals like iron, calcium, magnesium and zinc, essential amino acids, and essential oils in the form of the omega fats. But, we don't need to consume them every moment of every day. As long as we choose healthy food options during our feeding window, there's no worry about developing malnutrition. Ample time exists before and after a fast to make up for any missed nutrients by eating nutrient-dense food. It should be emphasized, however, that while there are essential proteins and fats, there are no essential carbohydrates. That means, of course, that there's nothing essential that will be lost to our health, by saying no to a cinnamon bun or danish.

The How To and How Long?

There are numerous protocols developed that make use of intermittent fasting, ranging from brief time-restrictions to extended week-long, and even longer, fasts. The three most widely studied intermittent fasting protocols are alternate-day fasting (ADF), 5:2 intermittent fasting (fasting 2 days each week), and time-restricted feeding (Table 10.2). The Alternate-Day Fasting (ADF) protocol entails switching between regular days of eating, when food intake is as per usual, or ad libidum, and fasting days, when there is either low or zero calorie intake. While this approach has a nice rhythm to it—one day fasting, one day not—it can cramp your style depending on your social calendar and travel plans.

The 5:2 intermittent fasting protocol is a bit more flexible in this regard. It's similar to the ADF approach in that there are regular days and fasting days, but instead of alternating between the two, fasting is restricted to only two non-consecutive days of the week.

The time-restricted feeding (TRF) protocol involves a daily partitioning of feeding and fasting. It consists of an ad libitum food intake during a specific timeframe (typically about 12 hours), and a night fasting period (the remaining 12 hours of the day), following the circadian rhythm. Commonly, folks who follow this latter approach, do so for only two or three days, and follow a regular diet plan on the other days of the week. This way, fasting days can be longer than just 21 hours. This approach is more popular, since choosing just certain days to fast makes TRF much more flexible and sustainable.

As mentioned earlier, before embarking on any one of these protocols, it's important to start by having a prudent diet in place—one that is devoid of junk food and focusses on whole, unprocessed foods and natural fats, with avoidance of sugar and refined grains—as well as a regular exercise program, including both resistance and aerobic workouts. Once these are both securely in place, intermittent fasting can be judiciously incorporated, slowly to start with and then adjusted depending on your schedule and preferences. The key to any fasting protocol is making sure it fits your lifestyle and can be something you can make use of for the long-term. I prefer the time-restricted feeding (TRF) approach, choosing one or two days a week to have a fasting window (typically 16-18 hours). This method combines the nutritional benefits of feeding, including the health benefits of breakfast, for example, with the metabolic and weight-control advantages of fasting.

Successful intermittent fasting takes some planning. To start with, I like to choose a busy day in my schedule for fasting that includes a morning workout. This is partly because fasting gives me a bit of an energy high, which I like to leverage. As well, busy days act to distract me from any hunger pangs I may experience while fasting. And, since I don't need to fuss about preparing and eating meals, fasting frees up time in my day, so I have time to exercise and get more work done. It's a win-win scenario—I gain time and lose weight!

When I choose my fasting day, I also ensure that I'll have ready access to plenty of water. Fasting while on a road trip, for example, is not a good idea. This is because if we want to fast well, we need to fast well-hydrated. For optimal kidney function, we need unrestricted fluids, especially if you're planning a workout during the fast. That means drinking enough water during the fasting window so that you are *aware* of your bladder—that is, you could pee if pressed. When you urinate during a fast, the urine should be pale straw-colored, and not dark yellow and malodourous. Although *dry fasting* (refraining from both food and fluids during fasting window) has been touted by some to accelerate the weight loss benefits of fasting, it's not a safe method and not one I would recommend. One way to make water more appealing is to drink mineral or carbonated water. My wife and I use a SodaStream system and carbonate our own water. It's far less expensive and avoids needing to recycle all those plastic water bottles.

In addition to plenty of water, I also drink black coffee and tea during my fast. This is because the caffeine acts to blunt my appetite and dulls hunger pangs nicely… and also because I'm a bit of an addict. I typically bookend my fasting window with a Doppio espresso (double shot, warm and brown, get 'er down), one in the morning, to wake me up and blunt my appetite, and one before I break my fast, to keep me going and counter the first-meal fatigue. During my fasting window, I sip on some black tea. I find the warm drink comforting and a nice change from the water. Green tea would also be fine, just no milk, sugar, or sugar substitutes.

Once you've got your fast day ear-marked on your daytimer, and water supply ensured, it's time to plan the logistics of the fasting window. This includes choosing a firm time that will mark the beginning of the fast, and making a mental note as to the finish time, depending upon the length of the fasting window desired. Then, you need to plan your post-fast repast. I like to break my fast with a cup of warmed bone broth followed by a keto-friendly mini-meal, typically a meat and cheese lettuce wrap. You don't want to plan to eat too much during the initial phase of refeeding, so you don't overstretch your shrunken stomach and suffer post-fast fatigue. As well, you want to avoid sugar and refined carbohydrates like the plague… or COVID-19, as the case may be. When we fast, our insulin levels are nicely reduced. The last thing we want to do is eat a Twinkie and cause an insulin spike, undoing our fasting efforts with metabolic mayhem. As Mark Twain said, "A little starvation can really do more for the average person than can the best medicines and the best doctors."

Days of Week	Alternate Day Fasting (ADF)	5:2 Intermittent Fasting	Time-Restricted Feeding (TRF)
Monday	Eat	Eat	12 hr
Tuesday	**Fast**	**Fast**	12 hr
Wednesday	Eat	Eat	12 hr
Thursday	**Fast**	Eat	12 hr
Friday	Eat	**Fast**	12 hr
Saturday	**Fast**	Eat	12 hr
Sunday	Eat	Eat	12 hr

Table 10.2 Popular Intermittent Fasting Protocols

Balancing Feeding with Fasting

"It all just sounds so complicated," Marion said in response to my fasting suggestion. "Besides, if I don't eat something every hour or two, I feel terrible. I think my blood sugar probably goes too low."

"Blood sugar levels can drop some between meals," I said. "But, since you're not on any blood sugar lowering medicines, I doubt this is the problem. Our bodies need fluids not food. Sounds to me like you're experiencing dehydration. It's easy to confuse hunger with thirst. Next time, try drinking a tall glass of water. It's surprisingly refreshing, and won't do any harm."

"I suppose I could try that," she replied. "But, this whole business of having an eating window and a fasting window sounds pretty difficult."

"Why don't you start by fasting between meals?" I said with a smile. "Substituting snacks with water would be an excellent way to prove that you don't need to be eating all the time. Then, you can try a 12-hour fast. It would give you some confidence in the process."

"I'm not sure I could handle the hunger," Marion countered. "All that stomach grumbling and panging. I wouldn't be able to think of anything but food the whole time."

"Hunger doesn't keep building during a fast," I explained. "Rather, it comes in waves. Drinking water and caffeinated beverages blunts hunger pangs, and appetite tends to decrease with fasting. This is because the level of our hunger hormone, Ghrelin, falls over the fasting period. It's not uncomfortable. I often even forget that I'm fasting."

"I don't think I'd forget," she said, shaking her head. "Isn't there a simpler way?"

"It's interesting," I responded. "Some dietary approaches, like the Keto Diet, sound straightforward—just cut out the carbs—but turn out to be very difficult to do and stick with, while other approaches, namely intermittent fasting, sounds challenging, but is quite simple to do. I think you'd be surprised just how simple. While intermittent fasting isn't for everyone, it is an excellent way to improve health and control weight."

Chapter Summary
Weight Control Fast

- The circadian rhythm regulates hormones, physiologic processes, and coordinates metabolism and energetics, including our weight control

- Disruption of our circadian rhythm is recognized as a risk factor for obesity and vascular disease

- Time-restricted eating can help re-establish our circadian rhythm and extend the benefits of sleep into our day

- Intermittent fasting can force fat metabolism and effectively reduce body fat

- The acronym, FASTING, lists some of the benefits of intermittent fasting, including Fat breakdown, Anti-inflammatory effects, Synchronization of circadian rhythm, Total cholesterol reduction, Insulin sensitivity, Normalization of blood pressure, and Greater energy and mental performance

- Resistance exercise is important to prevent muscle catabolism which may occur during times of fasting

- Patients with diabetes need to involve their primary care physician before embarking on a fasting protocol

- Fasting should be prohibited in childhood, pregnancy, and while breastfeeding

- Choosing busy days to fast can leverage the fasting energy boost, provide hunger distraction, free up time for getting work done

- To fast well, we need to fast well-hydrated
- Hunger comes in waves and diminishes throughout a fasting period due to the dropping levels of Ghrelin, the hunger hormone.
- Because the sensations of hunger and thirst can be easily confused, our first response to hunger should be to drink water
- Caffeinated beverages can blunt hunger pangs and help counter post-fast fatigue
- Choosing a keto-friendly mini-meal to break a fast can avoid stomach overstretch and fatigue, as well as prevent harmful insulin spikes
- Intermittent fasting sounds difficult but is relatively straightforward to incorporate into a healthy lifestyle of prudent diet and regular exercise

Chapter Notes

255. Dibner, C., Schibler, U., and Albrecht, U. (2010). The mammalian circadian timing system: organization and coordination of central and peripheral clocks. Annu. Rev. Physiol. 72, 517–549. doi: 10.1146/annurev-physiol-021909-135821.

256. Melkani, GC et al. Time-restricted Feeding for Prevention and Treatment of Cardiometabolic Disorders. J Physiol. 2017 Jun 15;595(12):3691.

257. de Cabo, R, Mattson, M. Effects of Intermittent Fasting on Health, Aging, and Disease. N Engl J Med 2019; 381:2541-2551.

258. Fung J, Moore J. The Complete Guide to Fasting: Heal Your Body Through Intermittent, Alternate-Day, and Extended Fasting. Victory Belt Publishing © 2016.

259. Anton S.D.et al. Flipping the metabolic switch: Understanding and applying the health benefits of fasting. Obesity. 2017;26:254–268.

260. Di Francesco A, Di Germanio C, Bernier M, de Cabo R. A time to fast. Science 2018;362:770-775.

261. Mattson, M. Intermittent Metabolic Switching, Neuroplasticity and Brain Health. Nat. Rev. Neurosci. 2018, 19, 63–80.

262. Horne B.D. et al. Intermountain Heart Collaborative Study Group Relation of Routine, Periodic Fasting to Risk of Diabetes Mellitus, and Coronary Artery Disease in Patients Undergoing Coronary Angiography. Am. J. Cardiol. 2012;109:1558–1562.

263.Sutton E, et al. Early Time-Restricted Feeding Improves Insulin Sensitivity, Blood Pressure, and Oxidative Stress Even without Weight Loss in Men with Prediabetes. Cell Met Vol 27, Issue 6, 5 June 2018, 1212-1221.e3.

264. Longo VD, Mattson MP. Fasting: molecular mechanisms and clinical applications. Cell Metab 2014;19:181-192.

265. Johnson JB, Summer W, Cutler RG et al . Alternate day calorie restriction improves clinical findings and reduces markers of oxidative stress and inflammation in overweight adults with moderate asthma. Free Radic Biol Med 2007;42:665–674.

266. Bhutani, S. Improvements in Coronary Heart Disease Risk Indicators by Alternate-Day Fasting Involve Adipose Tissue Modulations. Obesity. 2010 Nov;18(11):2152-9.

267. Hooper LV, Macpherson AJ. Immune adaptations that maintain homeostasis with the intestinal microbiota. Nat Rev Immunol. 2010;10(3):159.

268. Linghao L. The effects of daily fasting hours on shaping gut microbiota. BMC Microbiol. 2020; 20: 65.

269. Zauner, C et al. Resting energy expenditure in short-term starvation is increased as a result of an increase in serum norepinephrine. Am J Clin Nutr. 2000 Jun;71(6):1511-5.

270. Grajower M. Clinical Management of Intermittent Fasting in Patients with Diabetes Mellitus. Nutrients. 2019 Apr; 11(4): 873.

271. Bhutani, S. Improvements in Coronary Heart Disease Risk Indicators by Alternate-Day Fasting Involve Adipose Tissue Modulations. Obesity. 2010 Nov;18(11):2152-9.

Closing Remarks

One of my preferred pastimes as a youth was thumbing through my brother's old *Marvel* comic books. I spent untold hours poring over their worn pages and enjoying the action-packed illustrations of unstoppable superheroes and dastardly villains—Pow! Bam! Splonk! Voo-rooom! And no comic was complete until I had spent additional hours studying the back pages, advertising sea monkeys, x-ray glasses and ant farms, as well as gag gifts, like hot gum, squirting flowers and sneeze powder. My favourite ad was the full-page one featuring Charles Atlas entitled, "The insult that made a man out of Mac." Being a late bloomer myself, I could sorely identify with poor Mac and I dreamt of becoming a muscle-bound hunk capable of punching the bully and winning the girl. The advertisement made it seem so possible. In the promotion of his 32-page illustrated book, *Everlasting Health and Strength*, Atlas promised that he could "make you a new man, too—in only 15 minutes a day!" Although I never did send away for my "free copy," the ad left an indelible message on my mind: the way to happiness was by physical transformation. Through my troubled teen years of merciless bullies and distant, immovable girls, I firmly believed the notion that all my problems would miraculously go away if I could develop my wimpy body into an Arnold

Schwarzenegger ripped piece of work. So, I drank protein powder concoctions, bought sand-filled plastic dumbbells, and regularly watched the *Ed Allen Show* on Saturday mornings, in the hopes that transformation, and maybe a little respect, would come my way... C'mon, God! Can't the geeks inherit something on this earth, too? But it was no use. Puny pecs and scrawny biceps remained my lot, and instead of morphing into Hercules, I remained a dead ringer for Pee-wee Herman. Perhaps, if I had been more diligent and followed the instructions of Charles Atlas, I could've been a sexy specimen in a Speedo, rather than a waif in cheap clothing. No matter. I'm over it now and have come to realize that happiness has more to do with the transformation of the mind than of the body, and that health—that highly coveted state of being—is far more complex than what's achieved by following comic book advice, and far more achievable than trying to tease a *Tic* of a body into a *Terminator*.

Few of us seem happy in our own skin. If we're not complaining about being too fat and out of shape, then we're grumbling that our noses are too long and pointed, or flat and flared. It's hard to be content with the run-of-the-mill reflection in the mirror when we're ruthlessly reminded of our physical imperfections by the highly celebrated Hollywood hotties. You can't even grab a jug of 2 percent milk and a few Granny Smith apples at the corner grocer without being visually inundated at the checkout stand by a barrage of magazine covers portraying scantily clad beauties. Even though most of what the models are flaunting is fake and the rest is creatively airbrushed into submission, their contrived appearances insinuate to the onlooker, "Roses are red/ violets are blue/ God made us beautiful/ what happened to you?" It's enough to give the most stalwart among us an inferiority complex. But, despite my low regard for pop culture magazines, if there's a lineup at the till, I invariably grab one of these rags off the rack, anyway, and leaf through it to pass the time. And in the course of trying to find that article about Michael Jackson and "what really happened," I pass over reams of advertisements peppering the pages. The "before and after" comparisons never fail to capture my attention. It's an effective sales gimmick used to profile so-called health and fitness products and perpetuates that lie about physical change bringing happiness. Since we can so readily identify with the sorry sot in the "before" picture, we become easy targets for the promises implied by the "after." It's no wonder so many of us buy into the myth of magical transformation—and why not? If Plain Jane made the change, why can't we? Why should we be content being a frog, when becoming a prince or princess is a possibility? The advertisements promise the extraordinary out of the ordinary: flatter tummies, leaner thighs, tighter buns, and better sex—"and don't delay 'cause there's a full money-back guarantee if you order today!" The problem is, of course, that these promises tend to be merely hype and hoopla, bereft of substance and brimming with baloney. We are like Hans Christian Andersen's Emperor parading through town in nothing but his boxers if we think any differently.

It's all a big business illusion, designed with one singular purpose: to swindle us out of our hard-earned dollars and keep the oppressive world of consumerism spinning round. We need to know that health, in general, and cardiovascular health, in particular, isn't achieved by some secret Houdini transformation act. There's no two-week tomato diet, secret cellophane wrap, or easy way gadget that's going to solve whatever weight problems we might be struggling with and make us more dashing, debonair, interesting, or influential. As Oprah Winfrey wisely observed, "The big secret in life is that there is no big secret. Whatever your goal, you can get there if you are willing to work."

Our health goals, especially our weight loss goals, need to be sensible. We don't have to boast a perfect body to be healthy. Cracking walnuts with buns of steel or grating cheese off sculpted six-packs might be handy if we happen to be making a fancy green salad and find ourselves out of utensils, but such physical feats are unnecessary for cardiovascular health. Chiseled abs might be considered the current badge of health by the marketers of the so-called beauty industry, but they are unnecessary to achieve and enjoy heart health. From a cardiovascular vantage point, it's not about superficial appearance; vascular health is worked out on a deeper plane. We need to concern ourselves more with protecting the lining of our blood vessels, turning off the inflammatory machinery within their walls, and reducing cholesterol deposition. To accomplish this we need to trim down some, yes; but instead of crunching out a thousand sit-ups a day or following some draconian diet, we can get out from under the grip of vascular disease by focusing on modest weight reduction. Studies indicate that reducing our body weight by as little as 5 percent can pay marked health dividends.[272] So, forget the Barbie-wannabe, taut and tanned fashion models; they aren't promoting the beauty of health, but rather some unreal caricature of beauty. Besides, Barbie is nothing more than an example of body proportion distortion. Truth be told, if Mattel's fifty-year-old Barbie doll, with her long legs, wasp waist, big bust and slender neck were scaled up to life-size, she would be over seven-feet tall; a towering Amazon, so unbalanced, she probably wouldn't be able to stand, let alone sway down the runway; and so thin she'd likely lack the necessary body fat to menstruate—a jaw-dropping one-in-a-million girl, maybe, but as for a healthy role model, not a chance. The standards of the beauty industry are anything but healthy. We all would do well to forget superficial appearances and consider the words of singer Jonny Diaz, who said, "There could never be a more beautiful you/ Defy the lies, disguises and hoops they make you jump through/ You were made to fill a purpose that only you could do/ So there could never be a more beautiful you."

Weight reduction is an important component of cardiovascular health, to be sure. Obesity is related to higher death rates and there's a growing body of evidence demonstrating that weight loss can significantly improve our long-term survival.[273] But it's not weight loss at any cost. We must be careful about how we go about losing those unwanted pounds. Cardiovascular health is neither a competition nor a sprint. Similar to how the tortoise beat the hare, slow and steady is the best approach for beating fat and will promise the highest likelihood of long-term cardiovascular health. So, relax. There's no rush to finish our weight loss efforts, only urgency to begin them. And, as we begin, we must keep in mind that fat—even the unflattering, inflammation-triggering abdominal fat—isn't the only kid on the risk factor block. There's a long list of brats running amuck on our vascular streets, ringing doorbells and spraying graffiti, including high blood pressure, diabetes, elevated cholesterol levels, sedentary living, psychological stress, sleep deprivation, and smoking—it's a veritable block party from hell. While not all of these risk factors may be of equal importance to the promotion of atherosclerosis, they each play a role in vascular disease and deserve our attention, at least as much as weight reduction does. The goal of losing weight, therefore, can't be given a life of its own but needs to be incorporated into the larger framework of our lives, where we take into account all the risk factors at large.

The temptation to compartmentalize our lives into separate areas of work, leisure, socializing, hobbies, travel, and then a little "health" tacked on the side if there's still time, is a strong one. But this is wrong thinking and wrong living. Health is an attitude that must permeate every aspect of our lives—work and play, night and day. We must remember that the ways of enjoying life promoted by our culture—lying around on a hammock, eating a Happy Meal, or sipping on a Coconut Cream Frappuccino—are in defiance of our vascular health and we need to guard ourselves against them. Healthy living is an alternative to the dominant ways of our culture, not a supplement, and it's intimately linked to the many activities that make up our typical day. This includes what we eat, most certainly, but our health isn't limited to dietary matters. The *how* of health can't be reduced to a *how-to* dietary formula. All of the activities that we engage in throughout the day are important to our vascular health—drinking, walking, crying, laughing, meditating, and sleeping. From rising in the morning to retiring at night, our cardiovascular health is intimately linked to every aspect of our day-to-day living. So, rather than obsessing over "before" and "after" pictures, we need to give some attention to the decisions we make during the in-between times; the day to day; season in, season out; morning, noon, and night times. As Robert Pirsig said, "To live for some future goal is shallow. It's the sides of the mountain that sustain life, not the top."[274] Choosing cardiovascular health means choosing to make the most of the climb and not just grumbling and grunting until you reach the summit and can add your name to the metal box at the top. There's so much beauty around us to take in; it's good to stop and savour it awhile, and perhaps catch one's breath. Since good company on any journey makes the way seem shorter, our efforts at weight reduction and health maintenance will be more enjoyable and more fruitful if we involve those in our circle—our family, friends and community—and enlist the assistance of trained professionals, like personal trainers, dieticians and our family physicians. No dieter is an island. So, make your successful journey to heart health a shared one.

Chapter Notes

272. Lau DC, Douketis JD, Morrison KM, Hramiak IM, Sharma AM, Ur E; Obesity Canada Clinical Practice Guidelines Expert Panel. 2006 Canadian clinical practice guidelines on the management and prevention of obesity in adults and children [summary].CMAJ. 2007 Apr 10;176(8):S1-13. Review.

273. Rider O, Francis JM, Ali MK, Petersen SE, Robinson M, Byrne JP, Clarke K, Neubauer S. Beneficial cardiovascular effects of bariatric surgical and dietary weight loss in obesity. J Am Coll Cardiol 2009;54:718-26.

274. Robert M. Pirsig. Zen and the Art of Motorcycle Maintenance: an inquiry into values. William Morrow and Company ©1974.

Index

A

H

I

J

W

waist circumference **74-80**, 82-83, 106, 164, 195, 202-203, 317

Watson and Crick 34

weight cycling 201-203

Weight Wise Program 108

Welles, Orson 264

Winfrey, Oprah 376

World Health Organization 209, 309

Z

Zeitgebers 281